A CUP OF COFFEE WITH

10

OF THE TOP
COSMETIC DENTISTS
IN THE UNITED STATES

VALUABLE INSIGHTS YOU SHOULD
KNOW BEFORE YOU HAVE
COSMETIC DENTAL WORK DONE

Robin Rutherford, D.D.S.
Randy Van Ittersum

LEGAL DISCLAIMER

TABLE OF CONTENTS

ACKNOWLEDGEMENTS

We all want to thank our husbands and wives, fathers and mothers, and everybody who has played a role in shaping our lives and our attitudes.

To all the clients we've had the honor of working with, who shaped our understanding of the difficulty of this time for you and your families. It has been our privilege to serve each and every one of you.

INTRODUCTION

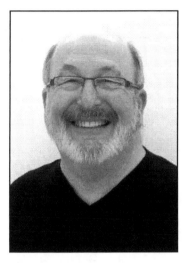

Contributing Author:

Randy Van Ittersum

Host & Founder – Business Leader Spotlight Show

Your smile speaks volumes about you. It is your smile that opens doors for you in the business and the social world. It is your smile that holds the key to all-important first impressions and, in many ways, dictates the way in which others relate to you. Your smile is one of your most valuable assets on the road to success in life. That's all well and good unless you happen to be one of the millions of people whose crooked, missing, discolored, or otherwise defective teeth cause them to hide their mouths when they speak.

ARE YOU GIVING THE WRONG IMPRESSION WHEN YOU SPEAK?

As many people with imperfect smiles will tell you, they often avoid the eyes of others when they talk to them. They frequently look elsewhere in an attempt to direct the gaze of the person with whom they are talking somewhere, (anywhere), other than their faces. They attempt to cover their mouths as they speak—casually, sometimes, with just a finger or two touching their lips or, more dramatically, with an entire newspaper or magazine.

We are generally unconscious about such "hiding" behaviors since we've likely been performing these maneuvers for years. We are also most likely unconscious of the fact that we are sending a terrible message to our counterpart. The message they get is this one: "This person has something to hide." "The person I'm talking to is dishonest." It probably never occurs to your partner in conversation that you're merely trying to hide your stained, crooked, and unsightly teeth.

How Long Has Your Smile – Or Lack Thereof – Been Holding You Back?

It isn't just prospective employers who sense your discomfort and evasive behavior. Before the internet, it was impossible for you to kindle a romantic flame because you were hiding behind your hands. Now that you've met the love of your life online, how will you actually greet this person in real life? Did you send him somebody else's picture? Oops. There's deceit in there somewhere, and a real relationship is based on trust. Once again your smile has cost you your share of happiness.

But what can be done about your imperfect smile now that you're an adult? It's too late for braces, right? Isn't dental work horribly expensive? What if you were to have cosmetic dental work done and still not rise quickly to the top of the heap at the office? What, you ask yourself, makes me worthy of that kind of upgrade?

Here's A Bulletin: You're Worth It.

In **A Cup of Coffee with 10 of the Top Cosmetic Dentists in the United States**, we offer the advice and experience of ten of the country's top professionals in the field of cosmetic dentistry. These men and women will introduce you to state-of-the-art techniques and procedures that can change your entire life in the space of one or two trips to the dentist's office. They will share stories of how improvements to your smile really can help you improve the other facets of your life. In other words, this book will help you understand that something CAN be done to level your own personal playing field and to give you the chance to score in ways you'd never imagined. You can eliminate some of the challenges you've faced and make a new start at a better, more productive and satisfying life. Yes, there is a cost involved, but you've paid the price for advantages before.

HOW MUCH IS AN HONEST ADVANTAGE WORTH?

When you went to college, how much did you pay for your degree? Why did you fork over all that money? You paid the price simply because you knew that such an investment would pay off in the future. Need we say more?

Okay. Perhaps you see yourself as "just" a stay-at-home mom. (A vastly underrated assessment, we're certain.) The children need shoes. The groceries and the mortgage eat up your husband's paycheck. Ultimately, in the larger scheme of things, your vanity doesn't count, right? Wrong.

First of all, put the idea of "vanity" out of your mind. Vanity isn't the problem here. It is your sense of worth that really matters. It is from your own confidence and grace that your children will learn to deal with the world. It is from your example that your offspring will develop their own style of interaction with others. Do you really want them to pick up your habit of telegraphing timidity and fear? Of course you don't. You want them to project a confident, winning approach to challenges. But how can they be fearless when you don't demonstrate a positive approach by example.

YEAH, BUT...

If you find yourself reading this introduction and muttering, "Yeah, but... my problem goes beyond whitening and chip-fixing," keep reading. You are probably aware of just a few of the procedures available today to improve upon the smile of just about anybody. There are whitening techniques in a number of different cost ranges. There is straightening by way of Invisalign® invisible dental alignment devices. You've heard of people resurfacing their teeth and/or replacing missing ones without the bother of bridges and partials. But did you know that if your wide smile reveals gums that go on and on, that can be fixed in a few short minutes in your dentist's chair? Were you aware that your receding gums can be made to look like they did when you were young, snug and pink?

WHY THIS BOOK?

Unlike many makeover books, **A Cup of Coffee with 10 of the Top Cosmetic Dentists in The United States** does not contain the kind of patronizing information that you might find in the latest edition of Cosmo.

Instead, it provides accurate information from the best cosmetic dentists about the newest products and procedures available today to literally change your smile overnight. And person after person will attest that going from stained, crooked, and missing teeth to a natural, beautiful, Hollywood smile will transform your life.

Here is just a taste of what you're about to discover:

- What to look for in a cosmetic dentist to practically guarantee you will get the smile you desire.

4

- Which whitening process you should use to get a natural beautiful smile.

- Which treatment option is best for you? Will the conservative options with minimal cost work for you? Or, will you choose the more complex options that require a larger investment.

- We will reveal how in a matter of two visits, you can have a complete smile makeover.

- And so much more...

A beautiful smile can transform your negative emotions into a steam engine of enthusiasm and self-confidence that will change the rest of your life.

Within the covers of this book, you may find solutions for the problems you've been burdened with for most of your life. And, while it's true that fixing your smile won't entirely fix your relationships or your career, it will give you more confidence and self-assurance so that you will better understand your own worth. Your new self esteem will carry you forward on wings you never knew you had. Most importantly, this book will help you to understand that with modern dental technology, a better, more powerful life awaits you.

Randy Van Ittersum
Host & Founder – Business Leader Spotlight Show

1

When Choosing A Cosmetic Dentist, Look For Experience And Advanced Training

by Robin Rutherford, D.D.S.

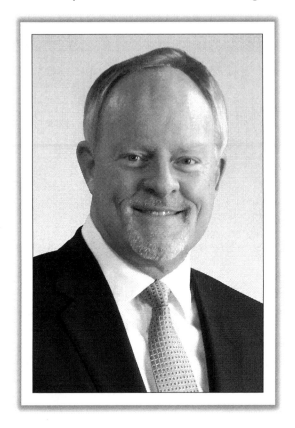

Robin Rutherford, D.D.S.
The Art of Dentistry
Odessa, Texas
www.gentledentaldoc.com

Dr. Rutherford is a member of the American Academy of Cosmetic Dentistry and the American Orthodontic Society. He is a Fellow of the Dental Organization for Conscious Sedation, an honor achieved by fewer than 2% of sedation dentists, and mentors other dentists in sedation techniques. He is also a Diplomat of the American Dental Implant Association, the highest level of recognition awarded to less than 1% of its member dentists. Dr. Rutherford has trained with some of the leading dentists and top experts in the fields of sedation dentistry, dental implants, and cosmetic dentistry. He maintains an extensive program of advanced study, attaining over 600 hours of such continuing education in the past 3 years alone.

Dr. Robin Rutherford continues to receive honors and awards for his work. He has been voted the "Best Dentist in Odessa" by the Odessa American Readers' Choice poll, he was featured in Consumer Research Council's "Guide to Americas Top Dentists" in 2004, 2008, 2009, 2010, 2011 and again in 2012 and, most recently, Texas Monthly magazine included him as one of the "Texas Super Dentists" from 2011 – 2014.

WHEN CHOOSING A COSMETIC DENTIST, LOOK FOR EXPERIENCE AND ADVANCED TRAINING

Many in dentistry, there are general dentists and specialists, but a cosmetic dentist is not considered a specialist. Examples of dental specialists include orthodontists, oral surgeons, or pediatric dentists. Specialists are not permitted to perform other types of dentistry. For example, an orthodontist performs all services related to braces but does not fill cavities or extract wisdom teeth. Cosmetic dentists are usually general dentists who have added the cosmetic aspect to their practices because they have a special interest in and talent for this area.

When choosing a cosmetic dentist, it helps to understand a dentist's training level. Having a D.D.S. or a D.M.D. degree simply means that the new practitioner has completed the necessary schooling to become a doctor. This young general dentist has learned the necessary skills and information to obtain a degree, but that does not mean he has equal practical experience compared to the older dentist.

New dentists may think that they are well-trained and have all of the information and skills necessary to help patients, but to have the judgment and to be able to perform all the technical procedures that are needed to change someone's smile takes years of advanced study. This situation is similar to the need for a heart surgery. If a patient visits a cardiac surgeon who has only been out of school for two to three years, he may be bright, smart, young, and well-trained; but he may have only performed this surgery about twenty times. Compare that level of knowledge to a fifty-year-old surgeon who has been conducting heart surgeries five to six times a week during the past twenty-five years or so. That surgeon has followed the latest break-throughs in heart surgery and has attended countless continuing education courses over the years to increase his knowledge.

A general dentist right out of dental school has a small amount of experience and knowledge in every category but is not a master of any category. Excelling or becoming a real master in any field requires a lot of experience and continuing education. To continually grow and learn, it's necessary to take continuing education courses from the "masters" in our field, dentists who have years of experience and knowledge in certain areas. You have to invest the time to fly out to the seminar location, spend a few nights in a hotel, and pay all of the fees. That's the price of getting good at what you're doing.

In Texas, dentists are required annually to complete twelve hours (about a day and a half) of continuing education to retain their dental license. That is just the minimum standard that is needed to keep the license. However, to excel, dentists need to go beyond the minimum standard. For example, I once attended approximately twenty courses within one year, which works out to one course nearly every other weekend. I wanted to work really hard to learn as much as I could, as quickly as I could. At one time, I completed over 600 hours of continuing education over a three-year period in order to learn more about several major areas of dentistry: implants, sedation, and cosmetic dentistry.

A really good dentist—or any professional—will put in the time and effort that it takes to increase his knowledge base and experience beyond the standard minimum requirements. Going back to the heart surgeon example, patients should want a surgeon who has advanced certifications and awards from people who know something about the subject, because this speaks to the surgeon's dedication and experience. Similarly, it's important to choose a cosmetic or general dentist who has practiced for some time and pursued knowledge on the latest technology and breakthroughs. This is a good sign that the dentist is dedicated to his patients and will give you the best service and results.

COSMETIC TECHNIQUES

Whitening (Bleaching): Today, patients commonly enter my cosmetic dentistry office to whiten their teeth. If you look at movie stars from a few decades ago, their teeth may have been a little crooked and not as white as today's movie stars, but with today's dental procedures we can do so much more than was possible back then. So, the standard for a "nice, bright smile" is whiter and straighter than it used to be.

For patients who want whiter teeth, there are a few different possibilities including a hydrogen peroxide solution for bleaching. This really does not hurt a tooth while it whitens. However, patients whose teeth are sensitive to fruit juices may also be too sensitive for bleach. It may not be possible with bleach to get the patient's teeth as white as they want. However, if your teeth are perfectly straight and you love them (but want them to be whiter), bleaching would be the first and simplest way to accomplish that goal.

There are two different approaches to bleaching your teeth: in-home and in-office. Teeth can be bleached in the office within about an hour to an hour and a half with the application of a more intense and concentrated version of the hydrogen peroxide-based bleach. Most of the time, our dental staff will also shine a light on your teeth about six inches from your mouth while you wear little sunglasses (like in a tanning booth). This will help activate the solution for a more intense, prescription-strength result as opposed to an over-the-counter strength. In an hour or so, you can walk out of the office with a much brighter, whiter smile than when you came in.

My office also offers a prescription-strength kit for patients to take home. We create a set of plastic trays that fit your teeth, along with a bottle of gel for you to follow the procedure at home. Put a small amount of gel in your trays and place the trays over your teeth for thirty minutes. Most people sit and watch television or read while waiting for the solution to work. This slower, gentler method of whitening works well for some individuals with very sensitive teeth who want them whiter.

Over-the-counter brands offered at local pharmacies and grocery stores are much weaker than the prescription-strength solutions. Commercial brands will bleach the teeth a little at a time, but the lower concentration of solution will take much longer to produce results. Many people prefer the idea of going to the dentist for an hour or so and walking out with white teeth, as opposed to spending weeks using the over-the-counter method at home.

For my patients who have composite fillings, I recommend that they replace the composite to get the best results. Bleaching is intended for enamel and not composite material. Since the composite is porous, the stains seep in thoroughly, making it impossible to remove the stains through the bleaching process. If the composite is not replaced, the patient's teeth whiten while the composites now appear darker and become obvious and can actually look like cavities between the teeth. I prefer to perform the bleaching process, remove the composite, and then match the shade of the new composite to the teeth after they are bleached.

Recontouring and Braces: My patients sometimes complain that their teeth are chipped, uneven, or too long. That can be fixed by smoothing off and reshaping (re-contouring) the teeth. This technique will change their appearance dramatically. This simple process does not require anesthetic and only takes a few minutes in the office but dramatically affects the appearance of the teeth.

If your teeth are crowded or your upper teeth stick out a lot farther than your lower teeth in an overbite, you might need braces. In a way, orthodontics is a form of cosmetic dentistry since the braces enhance the appearance of your teeth and your smile. While cosmetic dentistry is primarily viewed as a way to change your appearance, braces also improve the health of your teeth by aligning them so they fit together properly.

Cosmetic dentistry can certainly combine techniques, such as correcting tooth alignment with braces and then whitening the teeth that are now straight. As I previously mentioned, the orthodontist is only permitted to do orthodontic work and won't be able to perform the whitening procedure. By contrast, a general dentist can do as much or as little of all the different areas of dentistry with which he is comfortable and knowledgeable. This is one reason why the experienced and highly educated general dentist is in the best position to perform all of the various procedures needed to give you your most amazing smile. This goes back to my strong belief in continuing education, which allows me to perform a variety of services for my patients. While I am a general dentist, I have been installing full braces for thirty years in my practice. With this ability in my "toolbox" of services, I can do whatever is necessary to get the kind of smile that my patient desires.

Crowns and Veneers: Let's imagine that one of my patients has chipped or broken teeth or her teeth are a little crowded but not enough to require braces. Perhaps, she just doesn't want to spend a year or two wearing braces. It may be time to review porcelain veneers or crowns. Crowns have come a long way from the 1950s when dentists used silver or gold to make crowns. Way back in those days, you could easily spot a crown. In the 1960s, dentists learned how to cover the metal with porcelain to better blend in with the natural color of our patients' teeth. The black line remained, right along the gum line where the metal was visible, but the crown was much less noticeable even though people could tell it was there. Today, new generations of crowns are being used that do not need the metal for strength. All-porcelain crowns are so much more natural-looking and beautiful than porcelain-to-metal!

A crown is like a thimble. A thimble slips down over your fingertip and acts like "armor" to make your fingertip stronger and protect it from harm. In the same way, a crown slides down over the tooth and covers it to make it stronger while correcting any remaining problems with the tooth. Some patients say that they do not like or want crowns because they are only familiar with the porcelain-to-metal crowns that show metal at the gum line. However, when they see the new all-porcelain crown technology, they realize that crowns are an amazing tool in cosmetic dentistry. All-porcelain veneers are essentially the same thing as all-porcelain crowns, except veneers only cover the part of the tooth that you see—about three-quarters of it—whereas a crown wraps around 360 degrees of the tooth for maximum strength. However, an all-porcelain crown and a porcelain veneer look exactly the same. Crowns and veneers can be used to hide imperfections, lengthen the tooth, or widen the tooth. If the tooth has a large cavity that has been filled or may not be very strong, I use a crown to strengthen the tooth as well as to correct any cosmetic issues.

How Many Teeth Do I Need To Include? When I am working on a patient's front teeth, there are several things to consider regarding crowns and veneers. For example, let's say that you have a space between your two front teeth. It may be possible to close the gap by using veneers or crowns. If you have small teeth, closing the gap with veneers or crowns will look good, because the size of the teeth will be increased to close the gap. They will look normal. However, if you have two already-large front teeth (central incisors), adding the crowns or veneers may give you the appearance of having two large horse teeth. Instead, I may need to work on four teeth across the top (instead of just working on the top two teeth) to proportionately increase the width of the four teeth and fill in the gap without unnaturally changing the proportions of the teeth.

Anything done on the front teeth must match the color of the rest of your natural teeth or everyone that looks at your teeth will immediately know that you've had work done on them. Therefore, your first decision is whether or not you like the color of your teeth. If you do indeed want to whiten your teeth, I need to do that first. Then the veneers or crowns can be matched to the color after bleaching. Unfortunately, bleaching can be somewhat unpredictable. I don't absolutely know how white your teeth will—or will not—be after the bleaching process. This is because some teeth are easier to bleach than other teeth. For example, it may be easier to remove yellow stains than it will be to remove darker stains. If a bleaching treatment doesn't achieve the color that you desire, veneers can be applied to all of the visible teeth to give you the white color that you desire. The teeth in the back can probably be left alone, if they truly do not show, as long as they are strong and healthy.

However, having said all that, it would be a mistake to think that no one will notice your darker teeth in the back of your mouth. Consider how your smile will look from all angles and not just from looking straight into a mirror. When you are talking to people in a group, it is very easy to see someone's back teeth. I suggest that you look in a mirror and smile as widely as possible, then count how many teeth you can see. Then ask a friend to look at your teeth from the side and count how many teeth they can see. They will easily be able to see more of your teeth than you thought were visible. The number of teeth that show up when you smile your maximum smile will depend on the width of your smile, which is different for each person. Generally, about five teeth on either side will show; or a few more if you have a very wide smile such as the actress, Julia Roberts, has.

Gummy Smiles: Many people don't know about gum lifts, though this procedure isn't necessarily new. Have you ever seen someone with a gummy smile? They smile and you see a large portion of their gums above their upper teeth. With a classic, beautiful smile, the upper lip will fall just to the very edge of the top teeth without showing much of the gum above the teeth. Most of the time, a gummy smile can be changed. A laser can trim the gums back so they do not spill over the top half of your teeth. It's like trimming back Bermuda grass that has grown over the sidewalk and realizing that you actually have a nice, wide sidewalk. When my patients' gums are grown over the teeth, their teeth appear to be square-shaped, instead of appearing taller than they are wide as they should. In most cases, once we trim the gums, patients find that they have shapely, pretty teeth.

The Dental Facelift: It's tragic that many people casually choose to have any hurting tooth pulled. I find that patients tend to choose this with back teeth more than front teeth because they incorrectly think that back teeth are not as valuable as those in front. Unfortunately, now that you are missing molars, your bite will begin to collapse. You must bite down farther and farther before your teeth will touch so wrinkles appear as your face sinks in and you look much older. This also occurs in teeth grinding (known as bruxism). In this case the teeth are being worn down shorter, so your nose and chin get closer and closer together. A third example of this might be a patient with gastric reflux; having stomach acid in the mouth dissolves the tooth enamel and makes the teeth shorter and shorter. The classic caricature of a Halloween witch is drawn this way: a long nose and chin but with lips sunken back and nose and chin too close together, like a person without his or her dentures in.

A "dental facelift" corrects this loss of vertical height. Your teeth all need to be made taller to restore this vertical dimension and give you a younger appearance. By crowning most or all of the teeth, we can restore them to the proper height for that person's face. This causes the nose and chin to again be separated by the correct distance while also removing the wrinkles caused by the over-closure. In as little as two or three visits, you can look twenty years younger without undergoing cosmetic plastic surgery—which, without correcting the dental collapse, will never give you the results you are hoping for. Really, cosmetic dentists and cosmetic plastic surgeons (physicians) should work together on most cases of middle-aged people wanting to look younger!

WHAT DO YOU WANT TO CHANGE ABOUT YOUR SMILE?

When a patient tells me that he wants to change his smile, the first thing I ask is what he wants to change about his smile. Sometimes, what I think about what a patient should change does not match what the patient is thinking. One of my patients once wanted to keep the gap between her two front teeth. Normally, I would think that most people would want to immediately get rid of that gap. The patient said, "Oh, no. I have my grandfather's teeth and I want to keep that gap." Instead, she was thinking of other things she wanted to change. Once I find out what my patient wants, then we can decide together the best way to give her what she wants.

In consultations, I encourage my patients to take a long look at their smiles. If you want to take the time and pay the cost for cosmetic dentistry, you need to first make sure that you will be happy with the results. The actual procedures will depend on your unique situation, whether you need the teeth to be smoothed or whitened or wear braces for a year or two; or whether you need a gum lift or veneers on your front teeth or a "dental facelift" to correct loss of vertical dimension. Whatever you do, it's important for you to be happy with your decision. Smile as wide as you can and take note of each thing you want to change before beginning the process of cosmetic dentistry.

What's great about cosmetic dentistry is that it doesn't take a long time to change a smile. If you need crowns or veneers, the process only takes a few weeks from start to finish. You come into the office and I shape the tooth, making an impression to send to the lab, and place temporary crowns or veneers to protect the teeth while the lab creates the permanent ones. In two to three weeks, you come back into the office and I place the permanent restorations on your teeth. By the way, there will never be a time when your teeth will "look worse before they look better" because my temporaries will look better than when you walked in.

Implants: If one of your needs is the replacement of missing teeth, the best way to do that is often by placing implants. The implant is easily placed into a precisely-sized hole in the jawbone where the tooth used to be. It is basically the equivalent of the root of a tooth. A crown is then placed on the implant and the "replacement tooth" is complete.

Some people give up on their teeth and request that I pull them all and replace them with implants. However, if my examination shows that the gums and underlying bone appear to be a healthy foundation, I advise my patients against pulling all of those teeth to install implants. It would be like cutting off your leg instead of setting a broken bone. If it takes a few months for your real leg to heal, that's a better option than having to use a prosthetic leg for the rest of your life. A good and ethical dentist would advise that you fix your teeth whenever possible. On the other hand, if gum disease has eaten away at the bone and loosened your teeth, you may not have a good foundation to work with. Similarly, if you have a terrible decay problem and you have had repairs done, but the decay has gotten much worse or reappears every few years, it may not be worth trying to save the teeth. In this case, you may need to have several teeth replaced. In a worst-case scenario, you may need to have all of the teeth pulled and replace them with dentures.

Dentures with Implants: Dentures can be considered cosmetic dentistry since they can improve your appearance. When I replace teeth with natural-looking, attractive dentures, I am helping my patients improve their smiles. However, dentures do have their own set of problems and issues. The most common problem that I encounter is when a patient says they do not have any "grip" with the dentures. Usually, upper dentures stay in place because of the natural suction from the roof of the mouth. Some patients have a little problem with upper denture slippage. A small amount of denture adhesive usually corrects the issue. With lower dentures, however, you never get suction because it is just not possible with the tongue and lips moving up and down. The classic problem with lower dentures is that patients cannot "keep them still" in their mouths and start to hate the dentures because they can't eat with the dentures wiggling around.

Resorption is another denture problem that occurs when the gums and bone shrink away over time. The ridge (the horseshoe-shaped hump of your lower jawbone) is what the denture sits on and attempts to hold onto. If it has shrunken down almost flat the denture can no longer get a grip on it and so the denture skates around in your mouth as if it is on ice. To correct this problem, implants provide a stabilizing anchor for the dentures. By placing a couple of implants in both the upper and lower gums, we can create new dentures that snap onto the implants. This prevents the dentures from moving around in your mouth.

However, if a patient tells me that they cannot stand the thought of anything "removable" in their mouth—usually due to a strong gag reflex—there are ways to give them what they want without using dentures. We may be able to insert six to eight implants in the lower jaw, and four to six on the top, and attach permanent bridges and crowns to fill in between the implants. Therefore you can have false teeth that are not removable like dentures. For this procedure, get a dentist who has advanced expertise in this type of work. Again, this is where continuing education and years of experience are essential.

CONSCIOUS SEDATION MAKES FEAR AND ANXIETY GO AWAY

While all of these procedures are great, one of a dentist's greatest obstacles is a patient's fear of going to the dentist. Most people have good reason for their fears, such as a bad past experience in which they experienced pain. Some people may be claustrophobic—the thought of lying down in a chair with someone working so closely over them is overwhelming—while others may have a strong gag reflex. The result is the same: going to the dentist is very, very uncomfortable and scary for them. With conscious sedation, I can make all of this fear and anxiety go away.

One classic example may be a patient in her 40s or 50s who knows that she needs several root canals, crowns, or implants, but is afraid of having the work done because of her painful experience at fifteen years of age. She truly wants to have her treatment done, and now that her children are out of school and she has achieved a level of success in her career, she can afford to have the dental work done, but previously her fear made it impossible. Now, with conscious sedation, she does not need to be afraid or anxious.

Some offices choose to use pills while others prefer an IV to administer the medication. Either way, this medication does not put our patients to sleep, unlike general anesthesia used in hospitals for operations. Conscious sedation allows my patients to respond to my instructions (for example, "open wide") but they are not fully aware of what is going on. In most cases, they do not remember the work that we did after the medicine wears off. With conscious sedation, I can do any treatment without the patient feeling anxious and can keep the patient for a longer time. Instead of a patient coming back to the office two or three times to work on several problems, I can combine the work into one appointment while the patient is sedated. My patients do not need to miss as much time from work or their normal routines because we can do more at one time.

Conscious sedation is one of the greatest advancements in dentistry in the past fifteen to twenty years. I started doing sedation procedures around fifteen years ago. Since then, patients have constantly mentioned their previous bad experiences before they were able to get everything done through sedation, which has been a huge relief for them.

COSMETIC DENTISTRY CAN CHANGE YOUR LIFE

Anyone can be a good candidate for cosmetic dentistry if he wants to change his smile. Some common examples are patients wanting to change their smiles for specific reasons, such as sales professionals who meet with people to negotiate a sale or new business owners who will be meeting with many people and potential clients. They may want to change their smiles to enhance their confidence and appearance. To these people, cosmetic dentistry is a business investment. This also applies to people who are advancing in their careers, taking on a supervisory position or representing the company to other companies at conferences, and they want their teeth to look better. They know that their teeth are holding them back. It could really make a difference in helping them look more successful, like the kind of people that others want to do business with.

Some of my patients have been recently divorced and are re-entering the dating scene. Since they will be meeting new people, they want to change their smiles or take care of dental problems that they have been avoiding, usually along with losing weight or getting into better physical shape. Some people reach their 50s and realize they have been taking care of everyone else but themselves, from the kids to their elderly parents. They want to get their teeth fixed now that their children are grown and their lives are not as hectic. I've heard this many times: "Now, it's my turn."

One of my patients was a forty-five-year-old artist who came to me because her teeth were hurting. She traveled to craft and art shows to sell her artwork. She had stopped going to the shows because she was uncomfortable talking to people due to the appearance of her teeth. We began the process of fixing her teeth. Just after we installed the temporaries on her teeth, she went to a show and sold two paintings and a bronze figure. She was just so happy that she was able to re-enter life with new confidence. I keep photographs of some of my patients around my office. In her picture, she has a broad smile on her face as she is surrounded by an array of her paintings and bronzes.

A couple of years ago, my office held a contest for a free cosmetic dental makeover. Contestants submitted short one-minute videos explaining why they wanted the makeover. We chose four finalists who would have dramatic before-and-after results and allowed people to vote for their favorite. The winner was a single mother in her early thirties with two kids. One of her children has special needs and she wanted to go back to school and become a special education teacher. However, she did not feel confident in her smile or teeth, so we did a complete dental makeover. She went back to school and is now a special education teacher. It was wonderful to give her the confidence to follow her dreams.

I find that people who did not like their smile or their teeth often have to be encouraged to show their new, beautiful smile after we have corrected it because they have been subconsciously hiding their teeth for so many years that they have formed habits like keeping their lips together when they smile, ducking their head down when they laugh, or simply avoiding laughing altogether. When you know you don't like the looks of your teeth, it changes your personality. It's like going to a grocery store when you know your hair is a mess, hoping that you won't see anyone that you know, and feeling like you have to duck into the next aisle to avoid having them see you. Over the years, I must have seen a hundred people put their hands over their mouths when they smile or laugh. These people don't even realize that they have been covering their teeth or avoiding smiling because it's been a habit for so long.

Because of what we can do for people today, I think dentistry is an excellent area of medicine to enter. Any time that I speak with children or teenagers who say that they want to become doctors, I encourage them to think seriously about the field of dentistry. Dentistry is a branch of medicine and a dentist is just as much a "doctor" as is a physician. "D.D.S." stands for "Doctor of Dental Surgery" and "D.M.D." stands for "Doctor of Dental Medicine". These are exactly the same degree awarded upon completion of dental school but the various dental schools in different areas of the country choose which name to call their degree. It takes four years of college plus four very demanding and difficult years of dental school to get that degree, just as it does to get the "M.D." (Doctor of Medicine) degree. Doctors in each area of medicine specialize in their own fields without being able to do everything. For example, a cardiologist is not a dermatologist and a dermatologist cannot deliver babies, etc. Dentists deal with the growth and development of the face and mouth and the treatment of diseases and repair of damages to that area. As doctors, dentists are able to change people's lives and give them back their self-esteem and confidence. I love what I do, and I love that cosmetic dentistry is such an interesting and rewarding area of medicine.

When Choosing A Cosmetic Dentist, Look
For Experience And Advanced Training

(Disclaimer: It is only coincidental that Robin Rutherford, D.D.S. and Rutherford Publishing House have a common name. There is no relationship between the two entities.)

(This content should be used for informational purposes only. It does not create a doctor-patient relationship with any reader and should not be construed as medical advice. If you need medical advice, please contact a doctor in your community who can assess the specifics of your situation.)

2

BEAUTY—
STILL IN THE EYES
OF THE BEHOLDER

by Dennis J. Wells, D.D.S.

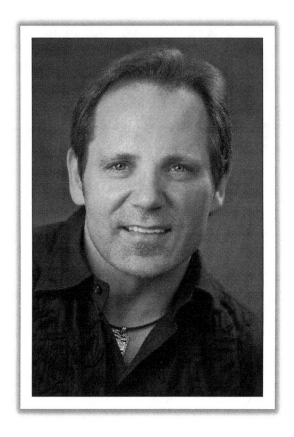

Dennis J. Wells, D.D.S.
Nashville Center for Aesthetic Dentistry
Nashville, Tennessee
www.drdenniswells.com

Dr. Wells has been a featured dentist on Extreme Makeover, the Learning Channel and Wellness Hour. Due to his exceptional work in the field of cosmetic dentistry, Dr. Wells was chosen as a "Top Dentist in America" in 2005 and 2010. In addition to his work in his dental practice, Dr. Wells is an advocate for others and is an active participant in several charities including Smiles for Life, Give Back a Smile, Dustin J. Wells Foundation, Smiles for Hope and Interfaith Dental Clinic.

Dr. Wells owns and operates the Nashville Center for Aesthetic Dentistry in Brentwood, Tennessee. Dr. Wells has over 25 years of experience helping his patients achieve the smile that they have always wanted. He is currently a member of the American Academy of Cosmetic Dentistry accreditation review board.

Dr. Wells invented and developed DURAthin veneers—the no-drill dental veneers that preserve more of the natural teeth. He instructs other dentists through seminars and hands-on programs on various aspects of cosmetic dentistry. He regularly lectures about cosmetic dentistry to impart his wisdom and knowledge to other dentists as well as networking with some of the leading cosmetic dentists in the world.

BEAUTY—STILL IN THE EYES OF THE BEHOLDER

The concept of beauty is subjective... and elusive. We each have a definition of our own. Among the most challenging things I do every day as a cosmetic dentist is to try to determine exactly what the consumer really wants to change about their smile and what their concept of beauty really is. Historically, in our field of dentistry, we have treated people who have been looking for what has been labeled the "Hollywood smile." Ironically, this term now seems to be somewhat irrelevant. You might notice that today, on television or on the silver screen, a lot of the actors and actresses and other celebrities—David Letterman and Jay Leno, for example—don't have the typical "perfect smile." Their smiles have characteristics that keep them looking completely natural.

Interestingly, there has been a push back within the American culture, perhaps beginning with some celebrities, against overly-corrected, contrived-looking smiles. People are migrating toward something much more natural and much more consistent with what we like to call natural beauty. We've all seen this played out in other facets of our appearance, from faded, torn jeans being in vogue as opposed to the starched slicked-out jeans that we've seen in the past. We've seen hair-styles go from being very neat and combed with gel to being messier and a little looser.

In my practice today, I still have people who come in wanting what I would call "fashion dentistry." They are looking for teeth that are perfectly straight and symmetrical, uniformly bright, opaque white, with no visible inconsistencies or flaws. More often, though, I have people who come to me wanting something very different. Their goal is to have a smile that looks like it grew there; not something that looks too perfect or artificial. To be honest, these are the smiles I enjoy designing most. I feel that emulating natural beauty with contours, colors and slight imperfections can be immensely rewarding both for myself and for my clients.

To figure out what each person wants can be very challenging. Being able to understand each individual's personality can help us catch sight of how their perspectives can influence their perception of beauty. I think, when it comes to beauty, it is certainly in the eye of the beholder. In addition to the clinical, health, and functional aspects of what we do, cosmetic dentistry is a form of visual art. Much like art, smile design can be very subjective. Just as some would view a Picasso work of art and be innately drawn to it, others might not be able to relate to it as being beautiful at all. We dentists have the challenge, and sometimes the burden, of trying to understand whom we're serving on any given day. We must try to get into their minds and understand what their definitions of beauty really are and what they want for their smile.

Sometimes the patient doesn't know what they want and we have to discover it together. Of course, we encourage patients to look at photographs that give us a sense of how they define "beauty" in a smile. We also have great digital imaging software that can give us some sense of how different types of smiles would look as part of their face, but the best tool I routinely use to accomplish this is what we call custom composite prototypes. With these, we can take composite materials to simulate the smile design by creating prototypes in the patient's mouth. These temporary prototypes can be "test driven" for several days or weeks to determine if this is exactly what is desired.

We have found that nothing compares to being able to place a three-dimensional simulation inside the patient's own lips so that he or she can experience the look for a period of time. This way, one can get accustomed to seeing oneself differently and also get feedback from friends and family before the lab starts developing the final restorations. Once the "blueprint" is approved, it becomes a matter of having our lab recreate the prototype design and giving the patient what they have already approved.

Beauty is always in the eye of the beholder, and every patient will have a different take on precisely what he or she is looking for. I can't imagine serving the wide variety of patients we do without being able to offer them some method of test-driving a new smile. It is truly the best form of communication I have found.

HOW TO FIND *YOUR* COSMETIC DENTIST

It is definitely challenging for consumers to find the perfect match for themselves when it comes to a dentist—and especially a cosmetic dentist. Our work is done in such a sensitive area to begin with and is in a very personal space. Add to that the fact that the doctor will potentially be changing your smile – a very important part of yourself and how you present yourself to others. It's crucial that you feel you can totally trust him or her. It is also important that you feel comfortable with the entire team supporting that dentist. They will be your liaisons with the dentist and will provide the amenities and services that can help deliver your care in a relaxed, trusting environment.

One of the first points to drive home on this subject is that if you have a high level of expectation in regards to aesthetics (your appearance and how others perceive you), and this is something very important to you, then I think your challenge is to really seek out a dentist who clearly has the same level of focus and passion for appearance-related dentistry that you do. How do you do that? Obviously, the first thing you look at is their training and credentials. No matter how passionate a professional dentist may be about aesthetics, if he or she has no advanced training in this approach, then he/she is probably not going to have the competency level you need. Cosmetic dentistry is very, very challenging for many reasons. Someone with a high level of understanding of the clinical aspects of dentistry, combined with the visual nuances that go into detailed smile design, is sometimes hard to find.

Dental schools do not traditionally teach a great deal about cosmetic dentistry. They focus more on the other aspects of addressing dental disease and function. For the most part, knowledge about cosmetic restorations must be sought out by the dentist individually after completing dental school. When seeking a cosmetic dentist, you need to learn about what he or she can deliver in terms of their expertise. How much training have they had? How long has this dentist been practicing? Have they been keeping up with new technology and fashion trends? On top of all that, even if all things were equal, there is the matter of his or her artistic talents and other gifts they can bring to the table. One of the ways to see that is to view examples of their work. Any serious cosmetic dentist will have photographs of their work and can share them with you to give a sense of how they approach their work. Just ask.

It is important for consumers to know that at this time, cosmetic dentistry is not a recognized specialty within the American Dental Association (ADA). They did recognize many years ago, for example, that in order to do orthodontics, you would need more than the usual four-year program. Orthodontists must, therefore, go through another two- to three-year graduate program after completing dental school. Other specialties in dentistry, like oral surgery, endodontics, and periodontics, have similar kinds of requirements. However, a young dentist could graduate from dental school with the basic training and put a sign on the door right away that says he does cosmetic dentistry.

If you're interested in high-level cosmetic dentistry, you need a dentist who has spent a lot of time in training. You should be able to see those credentials visible on his or her website. It is also possible for you to discover, through a little bit of research, where they had additional cosmetic training, and what they have done post-graduation in the world of cosmetic dentistry. That research might be as simple as making a phone call to the office asking these very questions. It's your smile. It's worth the extra effort.

Another part of the process of finding a truly excellent cosmetic dentist is to look at the amount of experience he or she has had in this area. There are some gifted people out there who are clearly able to push through post-graduate training quickly, and within a relatively short period of time, acquire a lot of knowledge. But, in general, there's no substitute for doing hundreds or thousands of cases. You learn a lot with each case you complete. We use the term "practice" in dentistry for a very good reason. Designing smiles is always challenging, and there is no substitute for experience. The human body and the emotional aspects of changing a person's smile are uniquely different from person to person, and so there is never a time when you can honestly say you've done it all, or truly mastered the process.

There's another reality we cannot ignore in this field. We each have some of degree of innate artistic ability. We have some degree of ability to envision a project from start to finish. What I really find fascinating is this: I learn a lot from interior designers. The good ones have this incredible ability, this uncanny gift, which enables them to see a room finished before it's even started. They see the finished product in their mind's eye. And I think dentistry is similar, in that we need to be able to conceptualize the end before we even start the process. It's this skill or gift that will be the most difficult for you, as a consumer, to uncover by looking at a dentist's credentials or his advertisements. You're probably going to have to do more research. It helps to find other patients with situations similar to yours whose end results you like. Of course, word of mouth (no pun intended!) is always the best kind of referral.

It bears mentioning that in my opinion, any world-class cosmetic dentist relies on his/her patients becoming "raving fans" who tell others about their experience. In my mind, this is because I am in most cases striving to create results that are undetectable and look naturally beautiful. Therefore, you might not even notice that your friend or co-worker had their smile "done". More often than not, the results of our work are more subtle enhancements. In fact, with the materials and techniques available today it is possible to create restorations that even well trained dentists cannot detect from normal viewing distances – now that is exciting!

The most flattering compliment to me is when a dental colleague seeks our services for designing his or her smile. That might be one little pearl of information that will help you as you search. Ask another dental professional where they would have their smile "made over". As you interview cosmetic dentists, ask them if they have ever designed the smiles of other dental professionals. Many times, you can see examples of their work on members of their own team. Having the chance to see the work in person can certainly be helpful.

It is extremely challenging for a consumer to work through the gamut of difficulties and come out, through some magical intervention, with a good match. As somebody who has been in the profession a long time, I've seen very frustrating scenarios play out, with people who had a high level of cosmetic expectation being matched up with someone who has spent very little time focusing on cosmetic dentistry and in the end, the consumer walked away dissatisfied, and so did the dentist. Ultimately, it becomes a lose/lose experience for everyone concerned.

I personally believe that most dentists out there have a ton of skill and ability; otherwise, they would never have gotten through dental school. Nevertheless, I also believe that lining up with a cosmetic dentist means finding someone who has a similar vision, a similar personality, and a similar approach to life and its problems as you do. For me, it all boils down to a partnership based on trust. That's why it's always such an honor when a patient seeks us out based on someone else's recommendation.

There are numerous organizations in dentistry that share the goal of promoting the training, the education, and the ongoing excellence of dentists who want to excel in cosmetic dentistry. One of these organizations, in particular, has made an incredibly important impact upon my career. The American Academy of Cosmetic Dentistry (AACD) is the largest and strongest organization of its type in the world. This organization is completely devoted to promoting and to creating excellence and interaction with other like-minded professionals. They have a very well-respected credentialing system, and they also have an accreditation award that is given to dentists who have demonstrated their skills and presented numerous cases before a review board. This accreditation process normally takes two or three years to complete and is recognized by our profession as a highly distinguished credential. Consumers who are looking for a cosmetic dentist would do well to seek out a dentist who has achieved accreditation status within the American Academy of Cosmetic Dentistry.

AGGRESSIVE DENTISTRY VERSUS A MORE CONSERVATIVE APPROACH

We've traveled down many roads when it comes to theories and approaches in cosmetic dentistry. There was a period of time, in fact, back in the early 90s, when most of us dentists bought into the idea that we needed to take away a lot of tooth structure in order to create maximum aesthetics. Ceramic specialists, who typically build restorations for a dentist, generally prefer that we give them lots of space and room to work with. When a dentist removes a lot of the actual tooth structure, the porcelain layer can be thicker, which makes them sturdier and easier to manage on the models as the ceramists are building them in the lab. There is another component at work here, too. The manufacturers who produce the porcelains will guide the ceramists to stay within certain "minimum thickness" standards so they do not push the product's limits in strength.

While it is historically true that our ceramists like to have lots of space when they're working on dental restorations, it puts a terrific burden on them to replicate nature. The more that's been taken away from the natural tooth, the more challenge there is on the ceramist to create something that looks very natural, from the size and form of it, to the contour of the tooth, all the way to the optics of it and the way it reflects light.

With all the mechanics of building porcelain in the dental lab on stone models, ceramists might begin to lose sight of the patient's perspective on all this. For some people, if having a nice smile means drilling their teeth down a significant amount, they would rather keep their smile as it is naturally, albeit imperfect. For this reason, a more conservative approach to cosmetic dentistry has been largely consumer-driven. The problem is, if the dentist and lab ceramist are unfamiliar with natural tooth contours, the porcelain can look thick and bulky when the tooth preparations are minimal.

There is a very specific skill set that both the ceramist and the dentist must cultivate as they move through their careers. It is definitely more difficult and complicated as a general rule to create a beautiful case when you don't aggressively prepare the teeth. In other words, if we take away a bit of the tooth structure, it makes it simpler in some ways to make the contours more uniform, and it makes it simpler to get a more uniform color. A lot of the difficulty in creating cosmetic dentistry can be simplified if you grind down the teeth. We know this is true, because we've done it that way. Nevertheless, we now believe "less is more". So does the consumer, in most cases.

So there are definite challenges associated with thick ceramic teeth and many times we see outcomes that fall significantly short of natural-looking. In fact there are some iconic people out there in the media who demonstrate the kind of outcome where one's tooth shape and color doesn't look natural. From a form and contour perspective, this doesn't look acceptable, even to people in the general public.

The people in our dental profession who say they are against the more conservative approach—we call it prepless dentistry— are against it because they believe the aesthetics will always be compromised. They are going on the notion that if we don't take any of the natural tooth structure away, then it can be very difficult for the dentist and the ceramist to create the aesthetics we're looking for. This is because we are essentially just adding another layer on top of it with the porcelain restoration. To that point, it certainly is challenging to get results that do not look thick or bulky when no tooth structure is removed.

I never proclaimed this conservative approach to be easy. In many respects, it is harder and takes a dentist-ceramist team with a keen eye for natural contours. It also takes an experienced dentist who is familiar with the limitations of prepless dentistry, who can identify those areas that do not lend themselves to this approach.

Along our journey, we have discovered that about 50 to 55 percent of the time, we encounter people who have proportionally small teeth in relation to the size of the face and, in particular, the size of their lips. The lips are very important because they act as the frame for your smile. So, in our experience, about half the time there is a pre-existing need or desire to augment the size of the teeth. When we see these cases, they fit beautifully into this minimally invasive, no-preparation approach. One of the first things we ask a new client is, "What, if anything, would you like to change about your smile?" If they talk about closing spaces or making their teeth larger, brighter, or having more presence, there is a good chance we can explore the possibility of adding a customized layer on top of their existing teeth without doing any harm to their enamel.

There's a big distinction between minimal preparation and no preparation of the teeth at all. We prefer to do absolutely no preparation whenever possible. If we're not able to do that, then we drop back to our second choice, which is to do minimal prep, which involves a small amount of damage to the existing teeth. Many dentists these days are attempting to be more conservative. However, I think those of us who are stubbornly looking for methods that will create no damage whatsoever through prep-less restorations are still in the minority. Interestingly enough, this is what consumers want most. To them, even a small amount of enamel reduction is unacceptable, or at least something they would only consider if no other options were available to them.

So, about 50 percent of the time, we're able to go in and do these restorations without taking enamel away. There are very significant advantages when we are able do this. Probably the biggest upside of all is that the entire restoration is reversible at any step along the way. In order to give you an example of how important this is in our practice, allow me to say that we've had the luxury and the privilege of treating quite a few high-profile people with this approach—people who are pretty visible in the media. One situation comes to mind in which we had an "A-list" actress; somebody you see frequently in films and on television. She was quite concerned about how the results would turn out in terms of changing her appearance. We talked extensively to her about how we could fabricate the restorations without removing any of her natural enamel, and then, if she didn't love them, we could just take them off and she would be right back to her natural teeth again. We also are able to create what we call custom prototypes: hand-sculpting the smile design in composite material on the teeth as a preview of the design before we ever make final restorations. This particular patient was well-served by the prototypes. She was more than a little concerned that the media would note the change in her smile, and the internet scuttle-butt would begin. Our patient was able to "test drive" the prototypes to be certain that she liked the look and the overall aesthetic effect, and was certain that she wouldn't be creating a media firestorm about the "work" she had done. By not taking any of the natural tooth structure away, we have a reversible component to a smile makeover that is hugely important to many, many people.

Anybody we're going to treat will have some degree of sensitivity to obvious changes to their appearance, even if they are for the better. I hear all the time, "Please don't make my teeth look like Chiclets." And, of course, they give us examples of people—often celebrities—who have overly-contrived smiles. When people have this deep concern, our approach to not prepping their teeth, not doing any harm to their own enamel, along with having the opportunity to test-drive the new smile, really gives them peace of mind about the procedure. It also gives me, as a provider, the rewarding sense of doing no harm.

I certainly understand the stress and concern over big changes to a personal feature you've grown accustomed to in the mirror. As a provider, I feel an enormous responsibility that the outcome is excellent. Every new smile can create a ton of stress for me as well. By doing the prepless restorations, we can all avoid all of the negative pitfalls. I view this as the main advantage to doing the prepless veneers.

The second most notable advantage is that when we bond our restorative material, whether it is porcelain or composite, to the enamel, we have a result that rivals any other protocol in dentistry. Since we don't cut and grind the natural tooth, it retains its natural strength much longer. The structural integrity of the tooth is primarily provided by the hard outer shell; the enamel layer. The dentin underlying the enamel is not very strong, relatively speaking, when compared to the enamel. When we take away a good bit of the enamel as has traditionally been done for cosmetic restorations, we're taking away a good deal of the natural flexural strength of the tooth. That can cause a failure down the road; not only in the bond strength, but it can also lead to root canals and future instability, depending upon what remains of the tooth once it's been reduced by prepping. In my practice, we love to bypass all of those negatives by not drilling on the natural tooth. Therefore, we are taking the original strength of the tooth and adding another hard layer, thus fortifying it rather than weakening it.

The third advantage that we enjoy with the prepless approach is the natural optics we can achieve. When you do not prepare the teeth by removing tooth structure, one must be very careful to create restorations that are not over-contoured. You don't want them to be bulky, and this is one of the push-backs that many of the dentists have about prepless restorations. One company was working hard to promote this kind of restoration to the patients and the public. They were marketing the fact that there would be no drilling, no shots, and no pain. Some of the outcomes they featured were not very favorable—looking bulky and in-appropriate. We've been fortunate to work with a couple of top ceramists in the country to create these super-thin restorations that can look natural. The problem is because they are so thin, they're difficult to fabricate, they're difficult for the dentist to bond into place without having some sort of damage done to the restoration, and they are time-consuming to make.

But, once they're bonded into place, they're incredibly strong. I would compare it to a thin sheet of glass. If you have a piece of glass that's extremely thin and you hold it up without any support behind it, it's pretty easy to break that glass. But, if you bond it to a hard surface, then it becomes much more durable and far less fragile. Ceramic works the same way. Once it's bonded into place, it's very strong. In the end, if you are able to manage the bonding successfully, then the optics of the case can be extraordinary for several reasons.

One reason is that we do not have to recreate so much of the natural optics of the tooth. The natural optics are still in place and we're simply enhancing them a bit as opposed to recreating the entire structure as we must when we drill away most of the enamel. Since the restorations are very, very thin, they allow a bit of the look of the natural tooth to permeate through that restoration. This allows the light to play more naturally on the tooth. That reflection and refraction gives us optics similar to what occurs in nature. The restoration becomes an enhancement of what is underneath. From a cosmetic perspective, some of the best, most natural-looking cases I've ever done were accomplished with a prepless approach.

The last advantage for prepless dentistry is something I refer to as "tooth-banking". Dentistry has progressed amazingly far in the last 20 to 30 years. We have gone through an aesthetic revolution and we've learned so much over this period of time. We can use very powerful adhesives to place extremely strong restorations so that we no longer have to use metal. In the last 20 or 30 years, dentistry has evolved to a place where we are trying to use materials that replicate what we see in nature. While we're working in the right direction, who knows what dentistry will bring in another 20 or 30 years? By not removing tooth structure, we are tooth-banking. We are saving that precious enamel for future improvements in technology. Because we are not removing enamel, we are not closing the door on any future treatments that could come along.

This is critically important when we're working with an 18-year-old. We often find parents who bring in their young son or daughter who is getting ready to graduate from high school and planning to go to college. He or she is not happy with his/her smile and thinks perhaps it's holding him or her back socially or in terms of their confidence level. Perhaps the patient has what we call microdontia, where the teeth are just very small. With such a case, it seems obvious to me. We need to add more enamel-like material to create teeth that are a more appropriate size for the patient.

That young person has so many years ahead, and it is difficult to consider electively taking away otherwise healthy enamel. When the teeth are not diseased or compromised, it makes sense to me to look at ways to enhance the smile only with the most conservative methods. If we're able to offer procedures that will make the patient happy and confident, but do no harm to the teeth, then we can feel good about our part in preserving a patient's future options.

Knowing that the case will require a good deal of extra work and time, the ceramist and the dentist must first assure themselves that the additional difficulty and the experience we bring to bear can actually help us all achieve an excellent end result. Some cases have a more pronounced difficulty level, and we must reach back into our training and experience in order to meet those challenges. Even then, there can be frustrating situations. Sometimes you have to back up and redo things here and there to get the work precisely the way it needs to be. Is it worth the extra effort? Yes. I think this movement is slowly growing in our country and other areas of the world, including the European community, where they are embracing this minimally invasive approach in a big way.

Our culture, in fact, has been the most accepting of aggressive dentistry where we remove lots of tooth structure purely for cosmetic purposes. Other parts of the world have always been more resistant to that. I might add that for the last six or seven years, we have been training dentists in our office from literally all parts of the world. Dentists from across the country and around the globe come to our office so that we can teach our approach as we share the methods and the protocol for minimally invasive dentistry. It is satisfying to know that, in our profession, we are seeing a slow but certain movement toward dentistry adopting these techniques and moving away from the traditional, more aggressive dentistry.

As I have pointed out, there have been a lot of different approaches and philosophies in the field of dentistry over the years. I have practiced a lot of different variations of cosmetic dentistry and I see good and bad in all approaches. There is rarely just one answer to any dental problem. There are always going to be some pros and cons to any course of treatment when we consider how to make the patient's smile look better. However, the goal is always the same: to help the patient find the smile of their dreams. Over the years, in my office and in my practice, we have come to believe that the least invasive procedure is the best place to start.

MINIMALLY INVASIVE DENTISTRY

One of the limitations to using a prepless approach to smile design is when one or more teeth are rotated or positioned outside of the ideal arch form. Adding another layer on top of such a tooth would make it appear even more forward and too thick. If that situation exists, the dentist and patient must come to a decision; remove some enamel so the tooth appears to be in the proper place, or try to physically move it. When a dentist chooses to creatively find ways to achieve sensational smiles while still conserving enamel, they will constantly try to develop feasible ways to straighten teeth in order to preserve the enamel.

Because of the nature of our particular practice here in Nashville, we treat a lot of people in the music and entertainment business. Sometimes they have an extremely tight time frame if they are getting ready to do a photo or video shoot, or perhaps they just got a new record deal and they need that new smile sooner rather than later. In cases like these, we don't have time to straighten the teeth first. In those cases, we are sometimes forced to do some minimal reshaping of the enamel to redirect the contours within the smile. Of course, we would love to take the orthodontic path first, but many times we simply cannot do that and we're forced to go to plan B. The important thing is that our patient feels fully informed and we simply act as consultants; sharing clear, accurate information and allowing them to make the call.

When a patient can and is willing to do some intermediate type of orthodontic treatment, it really makes a lot of sense to do so. I will often encourage orthodontic treatment in cases where I think it is best for the patient. It certainly serves our mission of preserving the enamel, and orthodontia doesn't have to take years and years these days. Today, we have new and improved orthodontic wires, for example, that have a lot better memory that can move teeth more quickly. Add to that the fact that low-profile clear brackets and white Teflon-coated wires can be hard to see even from conversation distance. Some of these new approaches work to move teeth into alignment within months.

There is no debate that, in the perfect world, we would have all patients align their teeth orthodontically in the traditional, year and a half or two year time span so that all of the back teeth fit perfectly, all of the front teeth are perfectly aligned, and the chewing system is just absolutely splendid. However, we live in the real world where, many times, we're trying to improve somebody's aesthetics in a short period of time and do it in a practical way without totally disrupting their life. In today's world, dentists have several options for patients to consider. Sometimes, innovative technology such as Invisalign®, 6MonthSmiles®, and Inman Aligners™ can help move the teeth into a better position, thus allowing us to do very thin veneers and procedures that are much more conservative to create the final, beautiful outcome.

DENTAL IMPLANTS

There are many situations when we have the opportunity to help patients who have been faced with dental compromises, such as tooth decay, gum disease, and tooth loss. There are some people who have had the misfortune of being plagued with dental disease as a result of genetics, neglect, or a lack of under-standing about oral health. Some of the smiles we see have suffered as a result of trauma, automobile accidents, or sports injuries. Others have suffered a significant amount of damage as a result of excessive bite forces and grinding their teeth for years. These are the cases that sometimes require a more traditional approach in order to create the best possible results. With thorough and detailed diagnosis and planning, we have the opportunity to develop a "game plan" and help the patient move through stages toward restoring their smile from health, functional, and cosmetic standpoints.

Of course, in these situations, we still strive to create the best aesthetic end result. We still try to determine what that patient's sense of beauty really is and we still create prototypes that can serve as a test-drive for the smile. From these, we are able to create a blueprint for the laboratory to use in creating the final product.

Tooth replacement has evolved amazingly over the last 10 to 20 years. In this day and age, the implant has become an incredibly successful option. Not too long ago, if you lost a tooth, you were inevitably condemned to using a bridge which meant cutting down more healthy teeth to put such an appliance in place, or you would be forced to wear something removable that would snap in and out. Today we have a whole different story.

With tooth replacement by implant, the process is as close as we can humanly come to putting your original equipment back into place once you've lost a tooth. We refer to implants as "artificial tooth roots" and in our practice, we refer our patients to an expert implant surgeon for placement of the fixture. Once the implant is fully integrated in the bone, our job is to build the crown on top of it that will look like a real tooth. People who have implants tell us they feel even stronger than their natural teeth! There's very little downside to the implant process other than the healing time and expense to do it. The procedure is very predictable and is almost always our first choice in tooth replacement.

Bridges can still sometimes be a great second choice and, occasionally, if you already have badly compromised or damaged adjacent teeth, it can make sense to do a traditional preparation on those teeth and put a small span bridge in place. Long span bridges (where 2 or more teeth in a row are missing) are rarely used these days if we can avoid it. These kinds of restorations have traditionally had issues with longevity and if one part of a bridge is compromised with decay or fractured porcelain, the entire bridge has to be remade. We also have deep concerns about the negative effects of the additional forces being placed on the "anchor" teeth. In this day and time, we are more inclined to place implants where the missing teeth were. This allows the patient to floss between the teeth and also keeps the forces distributed on the teeth as intended by nature. Again, the important thing is that the patient understands all the pros and cons of each approach and is able to make a decision that fits him best.

So when people come to our practice with cosmetic concerns, we generally divide them into two basic categories:

- The first category would be the purely elective process, where the patient has very nice healthy, natural teeth that simply do not look as good as the patient would like for them to look. In those cases, we strive with all of our might to create an end result where we do little or no harm to the teeth, and hopefully bank that enamel for future decades and for the improvements that may come in dentistry.

- The second category is those people who present with teeth that have been previously compromised. Perhaps they have existing old restorations already in place, perhaps they've had tooth loss due to injury or disease, or perhaps they have some degree of trauma that occurred from accidents, sports injuries, or other things of that nature. In situations like these, we still look for the least-invasive way to correct the problem, but we are sometimes forced to move to more traditional types of dentistry. It is important to have a variety of approaches and techniques available in order to creatively develop the treatment plan that best suits each situation and each patient.

In terms of dental implants, there are improvements and advancements being made constantly. The world of implantology has exploded in the last couple of decades. Experienced dentists can now place implants with very predictable, positive results as far as a long-term prognosis goes. We're also able to create beautiful aesthetics with these, although it can still be challenging sometimes.

There is a debate raging today in the world of dentistry. When a tooth has had a root canal and perhaps a post and a crown, and has finally begun to deteriorate, at what point do we simply decide to take out the natural tooth? Should we place the implant and avoid the ongoing treatment? That debate will continue, I think. As we get better and better with all facets of dentistry, it becomes more difficult to weigh what we can realistically do to save a tooth against the option of abandoning that tooth and removing it. I tend to think that holding on to the natural root as long as possible makes sense. However, I have patients who would rather bypass the uncertain prognosis of infections, root canals, posts, and crowns and opt for an implant. I think either path can be acceptable, depending on the status of the tooth and surrounding bone.

As a consumer, you must be able to rely on the clinical judgment of the team of dentists who will do the implant surgery and the restoration to determine when teeth are hopeless and when they're not. You'll have to depend upon their expertise to know when it is time to consider tooth replacement with implants.

ABUNDANT REWARDS

Some of the reasons that I chose a career in dentistry were very superficial. I thought I could make a pretty good living in the field. I thought I could have my own business and maybe be in charge of my own time. From the time I was a senior in dental school, I realized that it was the artistic side of dentistry that appealed to me most. Now, after 31 years of practice—with three decades under my belt—I can tell you I've not been disappointed in my career choice.

When I was in my final year of dental school I was able to finish my credits early so I had a little free time. I spent that time working with cosmetic materials and doing things in the front of the mouth that people could actually visualize and could get excited about. I knew this was an area that was exciting to me and it was where I wanted to focus my dental career. I knew this was something that I could be passionate about. But at that time, I could have never imagined that the career I was headed toward would have such wonderful rewards. And they are rewards that are nothing like what I thought about as a young dental student. I never, in a thousand years, could have imagined that the biggest and most rewarding aspects of being a dentist—in particular, being a cosmetic dentist—would be the level of appreciation and the level of change that I could bring to a patient's life. This was something I had to experience first-hand.

Over time, as I began to have those opportunities and saw the ways in which changing someone's smile could impact not just their looks but also their entire life—the way they interact with other people, their career success, their degree of confidence—it was unbelievable to me! I came to realize that a person's smile is one way they connect to others. When we can enhance that ability, it has a positive effect in more ways that one. As my team and I got to experience that first hand, we gained a sense of deeper purpose in doing what we do. That sense of fulfillment continues today. Thirty-one years later, it is one of the biggest drivers that keeps me focused on why I do what I do every day.

On the subject of life-changing experiences, several patients come to mind. One young man in particular was battling a serious medical condition. He was a young man, still in high school and as a result of his illness, he had experienced dental deterioration, lots of disease, decay, and unsightly black areas in his front teeth when he came to us. He and his mom approached us at the time when he was getting out of school and about to enter the work force. He wanted to get a job, even though he was battling with his health. This young man looked at me and said, "Doctor, I do not ever smile because I am so self-conscious. I really think this is holding me back in all aspects in my life. What can you do for me?"

For him, we created a natural-looking smile, got rid of the black and dark areas, and he was transformed into a completely different young man. We not only changed the way his smile looks; we were able to change how he felt about himself. After that, he was able to go into an interview with new confidence and landed his first job. He was able to smile without having to hold his lips down to cover his teeth, and his life took a positive turn. We were able to do this in a relatively short period of time and the sense of fulfillment and purpose that brought to me and my entire team is hard to describe.

Here in "Music City" we also see young singers trying to make it in the music business, and by making positive changes in their smiles, we have been able to boost their confidence and help them to build a successful entertainment career. We've had young ladies involved with beauty pageants who were striving to win major competitions. We were able to create beautiful smiles that gave them the confidence that they needed to achieve their personal goals. We have found great pleasure in serving people from all walks of life as they embark upon the future ahead of them. Giving people the kind of smile that opens them to life-altering confidence and a new sense of joy has been, without question, the most rewarding part of being a cosmetic dentist.

(This content should be used for informational purposes only. It does not create a doctor-patient relationship with any reader and should not be construed as medical advice. If you need medical advice, please contact a doctor in your community who can assess the specifics of your situation.)

3

WHITENING REVOLUTIONIZED THE WAY PEOPLE VIEW THEIR TEETH

by Lana Rozenberg, D.D.S.

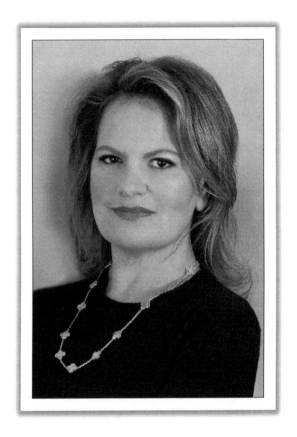

Lana Rozenberg, D.D.S.

Lana Rozenberg, D.D.S.
New York, New York
www.rozenbergdds.com

With her extensive experience in advanced dental procedures, Dr. Rozenberg is recognized as one of New York's leading cosmetic dentists. She is the creator and founder of her private practice, Lana Rozenberg, D.D.S., located on New York's Upper East Side. She serves as the cosmetic dentist to top editors of major beauty and health magazines. Her focus on the most advanced techniques in the dental field has led her to be featured in several major national publications and television programs, including Vogue, Elle, Harper's Bazaar, Allure, Health, Cosmopolitan, Glamour, New York Magazine, the Discovery Channel, Reuters News, Channel 7 News, NY 1 News, Fox 5 News, "Good Morning America," and more.

Dr. Rozenberg earned her doctor of dental surgery degree from the University of the Pacific Dental School in San Francisco, where she graduated in the top ten percent of her class. In 1998, Dr. Rozenberg graduated from New York University School of Continuing Education, where she received specialized training in Surgical and Prosthetic Aspects of Implants. She completed a mini residency in Periodontics at New York University the following year.

Licensed by the Northeastern Regional Board, Dr. Rozenberg is a member of the American Dental Association (ADA) and the American Academy of Cosmetic Dentistry (AACD). She served as a national spokesperson for Reach MAX Oral Care Products from 2002 until 2007 and as the spokesperson for Crest Whitening Products in 2010.

WHITENING REVOLUTIONIZED THE WAY PEOPLE VIEW THEIR TEETH

Numerous advances in dentistry have made it possible for people to improve or change their smiles. New technology and advances occur on a regular basis. For example, whitening revolutionized the way that people view their teeth. Dentists began offering in-office whitening services and that transitioned into a huge over-the-counter business as major companies began offering products that made a huge difference in a person's smile. With younger people who have minor imperfections, whitening can dramatically improve a smile.

There are several different types of whitening products, both in the office and over-the-counter. In-office treatments include products like Zoom!®, which whiten teeth in a dental office. Take-home products, such as whitening trays, can be worn by patients at night or during the day. Some dentists use a combination of the two procedures: whitening the teeth in-office and prescribing the whitening trays for at-home use to stabilize the color. Of course, several varieties of over-the-counter whitening products are available at your local drug store for at-home use. While over-the-counter products may not be as effective as the in-office combination for teeth whitening, they do still whiten the teeth.

Pre-existing dental work (e.g., crowns and bondings) is one factor that dentists look at when we consider whether or not a person is a good candidate for teeth whitening. Other than your natural teeth, nothing will change color in your mouth except for porous composite. If your teeth are discolored due to tetracycline or too much fluoride, they may not bleach very well, so it may be necessary to change the color of your smile with crowns, bonding, or veneers. Discuss the options with your dentist before you set out to whiten your teeth, especially if you have bondings such as crowns or veneers.

We all want pretty, white teeth that sparkle when we smile. My patients often tell me that they want their teeth as white as possible. However, there is such a thing as too white. Dentists gauge the whiteness of your teeth by the whites of your eyes. Since there are many different shades of white, if you have teeth that are whiter than the whites of your eyes, your smile will look like a flashlight, or like Ross in the episode of Friends when he bleached his teeth and all you could see were his teeth. A younger person will have whiter teeth than a 65-year-old person, so dentists will want to examine the whites of the eyes and find a color that looks more natural.

The other factor is the color of your skin. The darker your skin, the whiter your teeth will naturally appear by contrast. If you have a dark complexion, don't choose a super-white color because it will look even whiter due to your skin tone. For people with dark hair, I would suggest a more muted, natural hue of white compared to a person with grey or blonde hair, on whom a whiter shade would look more natural. If your hair is red, stay away from yellow shades—they will make your teeth appear more yellow. Eye color can also be a factor, although to a lesser degree than the whites of your eyes and your skin color.

The last thing that you want to hear is, "Oh, where did you have those done?" or "Whoa, what is that?" because that means your teeth appear to be fake. Your teeth should look real as well as beautiful. The best way to determine the color is to use a set of temporaries. It is difficult for a dentist (and very difficult for a patient) to look at a shade tab and determine the best shade of white. Due to current social messages, people want a super-white smile and will choose the whitest color even if it is not the best shade for them. A good dentist listens to and then educates his patient to understand that "toilet bowl white" will look toilet bowl white in the mouth. It looks awful and it looks fake. Good dentistry is about creating a natural, beautiful smile that compliments your face. If the color is too white, your teeth will be the only thing that anyone will see when they look at you.

NEW PRODUCTS AND PROCEDURES HAVE REVOLUTIONIZED DENTISTRY

I think the greatest innovation over the years were porcelain veneers (laminates). They are simply the best and most long lasting way to transform a smile in just two office visits. Veneers can correct many imperfections including changing color, shape of the teeth, making crooked teeth appear straight, correcting spaces between the teeth and giving a fuller smile by giving greater support to lips and cheeks. Porcelain veneers are thin shells of porcelain that are bonded over the natural tooth structure. They are as thin as contact lenses and very durable.

Porcelain fillings (inlays/onlays) is another wonderful innovation in modern dentistry. It is one of the most beautiful and natural looking restorations available today. It is an alternative to amalgam fillings (silver) or composite fillings. inlays/onlays have a high degree of strength and are excellent for function on posterior teeth. They restore and protect large portion of decay or under mind tooth structure. Unlike crowns, porcelain fillings only cover a portion of the tooth so they are much more conservative than crowns but very strong and durable and can last just as long. The process takes two short visits where the tooth is prepared, an impression is taken and a temporary filling is placed. At the second visit the permanent porcelain filling is cemented into the tooth.

Invisalign® another recent revolution has come from the Invisalign® products. Some adults who wore braces as children never followed up with their dentist, or didn't wear their retainers, so their teeth have shifted over the years post-treatment. As with most adults, they do not want to wear metal braces. Metal braces are still the conventional "metal smile" method of straightening teeth, even though they now include different colors and even clear brackets, because the metal wires running through the brackets are just as visible. Invisalign® revolutionized the way we think about braces, and many adults are embracing this as a way to straighten their teeth and change their smile.

First, the dentist will make a mold of your mouth and send it to a lab. The lab then digitally creates aligners that will slowly shift your teeth into their proper position. One advantage of aligners is that they are clear, so more adults are comfortable wearing them. The other big advantage is that they are removable. If you have a date, speech, or project in which you do not feel comfortable wearing the aligner, simply remove them and pop them back once the engagement is over.

Of course, one of the disadvantages is that a patient must be dedicated to wearing the aligners for the majority of the time prescribed. Otherwise, they won't get the desired results. However, the patient is in control of taking the aligners off and on, unlike conventional braces that are affixed to the patient's teeth and cannot be easily removed. By contrast, Invisalign® products do move teeth and move them beautifully. The aligners change an adult's smile, resulting in a beautiful and natural-looking smile with properly positioned teeth. If the patient has never had braces, Invisalign® is now available to him or her as a less invasive and costly option when compared to veneers.

DENTAL IMPLANTS

Another dental revolution came about with implants that replace missing teeth. Before implants, if a patient was missing a tooth or multiple teeth, the dentist would use a crown and bridge. If there were no posterior teeth to use as an anchor for a bridge, you had to wear removable dentures, which many people do not like or cannot wear without problems. Now, the dentist can insert a couple of implants to provide an anchor for a permanent bridge, which gives the patient the option of correcting his or her smile with a permanent solution.

CORRECTING GUMMY SMILES

Dentists also correct what we call "gummy smiles" with the use of crown lengthening. We remove some of the tissue and the underlying periodontium to elongate a tooth that appears shorter due to the gum growing over the tooth. The gum tissue is removed using a laser, while the patient is sedated under a local anesthetic. With laser therapy, dentists can remove the gum tissue covering a short tooth without any bleeding or much post-op discomfort because the laser cauterizes the remaining tissue. Afterwards, the teeth look much better because they are properly contoured with the proper dimension (so they don't appear to be too short) and the extra gum tissue doesn't show when you smile.

Dentists can also do a procedure called (lip repositioning TS). If your teeth are not short and they have the proper dimensions, but a lot of gum shows when you smile, lip repositioning can correct your smile. A small portion of the tissue on the inside of your lip is removed and the inner portion of the lip is sutured to the gum, limiting the muscles that raise your lip. By doing this, we minimize the amount of visible gum tissue. Unlike regularly applied Botox® injections, this is a permanent procedure, done under local anesthetic, which only takes about 45 minutes to complete. It does not change the appearance of your face but it does stop your lip from rising too high when you smile.

CORRECTING RECEDED GUMS

On the flip side, when a patient has recessed tissue, too much of the tooth shows because the gums have receded. The previous conventional treatment was to take a piece of gum tissue from a donor site, suture it over the recession, and cover the area of the exposed tooth. Most patients were unwilling to go through this procedure due to the discomfort involved. Now, dentists use a new procedure called the Pinhole Surgical Technique, also known as pinhole rejuvenation. Two pinholes are made just above the recessed area and an instrument is inserted into the pinholes. The instruments elevate the tissue from the periosteum, the tissue flaps down to cover the recessed areas, and then collagen is inserted to attach the tissue in the proper position. There is no need to cut a piece of palate from a donor site or use alloderm (a cellular dermal matrix); therefore, patients do not experience the usual amount of pain from the dentist's use of a scalpel and sutures. The procedure only takes about an hour to complete and involves very little discomfort for the patient.

The most recent dental advancements are seen with crowns, inlays, and veneers. Dentists can now use a CAD/CAM and scanners to complete the entire process in a few hours without the necessity of having two appointments and a temporary inlay, crown, or veneer. The traditional restoration process involves the dentist preparing the tooth and then mixing material for the patient to "bite down" into so that the dentist can send an impression or gummy "mold" of the restoration to the lab for inlay construction. Dentists currently use a digital scanner to scan the tooth so that a CAD/CAM machine can fabricate a restoration for the patient in about an hour. As a patient, you do not need to wear a temporary restoration and return in two weeks. You can complete the entire procedure in a couple of hours.

The restoration products created with a scanner and CAD/CAM machine are probably stronger and better than traditional products because of the massive amount of research that went into creating this process. Product development is a huge industry; all of the restoration products to the third and fourth generation are strong, and the bond is definitely superior than before. For the most part, veneers, inlays, onlays, and the porcelain restorations last longer because the products are so much better due to the research invested in the products' development.

Obviously, cosmetic dentistry has come a long way. However, unless the dentist is using the E4D CAD/CAM machine to create the restorations in-office, the restorations will be created in an off-site lab. Veneers are nearly always sent to a lab due to the higher aesthetic quality, provided it is a good lab. The lab must employ a highly trained lab technician who knows how to create restorations that look real and life-like. Even though dentists still use labs to create restorations, the turnaround time is much shorter—typically a day or two instead of a couple of weeks.

NONSURGICAL COSMETIC FACELIFTS

If your upper lip is too flat and your smile is too narrow, you may be a candidate for a "smile lift." The dentist uses a veneer or a crown to build up the teeth to reduce the appearance of fine lines around the mouth and to make the lips appear fuller. Instead of using Restylane® or other injectable fillers, you can use teeth for the same overall effect. Obviously, this procedure works on certain people but is not the answer for thin lips. Dentists must consider the entire shape of the face and other features because these have an effect on whether a smile lift will give the patient the desired result. It is so important to go to a dentist who is familiar with these types of procedures, because he or she will know what to look for and whether or not the patient is a good candidate for a smile lift.

More people opt for nonsurgical cosmetic facelifts to change their smiles rather than "going under the knife". To plump up their lips, people can get veneers or crowns to produce a broader, wider smile. The effect is similar to an injection because it fills in the area around the mouth and provides a more youthful appearance. Injections and fillers are not permanent and the patient must constantly get injections every six months, unlike a permanent dental smile lift.

In some cases, a dentist can make a trial smile or a snap-on smile to see what the patient will look like before the patient decides to go through with a cosmetic dental procedure. Veneers are costly and cannot be simply removed if you do not like how you look after they are finished, so a trial smile makes sense. Of course, there is a cost for trying the snap-on smile. However, because cosmetic dental treatments like veneers are not easily reversible, it is better to test-drive or preview the smile before you commit to the permanent work. A trial smile is something that I would recommend for patients who have doubts about the procedure. If a patient tells me that he/she is interested in having veneers but is not completely sure, test-driving a smile can allow him to make changes if he/she doesn't like the shape or the color of the teeth before the permanent veneers are applied. It is important that patients take the time to educate themselves about the work that they are requesting so they understand what is involved.

HOW TO CHOOSE THE RIGHT COSMETIC DENTIST

Of course, choosing the right cosmetic dentist is part of making sure that your smile becomes what you want it to be. For me, the two-part answer to "What is a good dentist?" is that he or she is qualified and that you feel comfortable with the dentist. The office should be clean, modern, and have state-of-the-art equipment. You should feel physically and emotionally comfortable so that you will have a good experience and be able to ask questions about the dentist's background and continuing education. The prospective dentist should be a graduate of a reputable dental school in the United States (check www.ada.org) and participate regularly in continuing education courses. Dentistry is an ever-changing field, so it is crucial that a dentist receive continuing education, especially in cosmetic dentistry, to keep up with the changes in technology and other advancements. A dentist must attend continuing education courses to stay on top of advancements.

Make sure that your dentist is a member of at least one dental academy, such as the American Academy of Cosmetic Dentistry (AACD). You can ask for a recommendation from the academy, though they do list all of their dentist members online. It is also a membership requirement that the dentist participate in a minimum number of hours of continuing education, so this is a good way to ensure that the dentist is staying up-to-date on new advancements. Since cosmetic dentistry is not an ADA-recognized specialty, cosmetic dentists are not required to attend continuing education to maintain a specialty status, but membership in a dental academy will hold the dentist to a higher standard for continuing education.

Some dentists refer to themselves as "cosmetic dentists" but it is not a true specialty like a periodontist or endodontist. Therefore, it is important to view examples of the dentist's work. Ask for examples of "before and after" pictures, and also ask about the number of these types of cosmetic cases that the dentist completes in a year. If the number is very few, that is probably not a good sign. Practice makes perfect in anything, so the more cases a cosmetic dentist handles, the better the dentist will become at performing those services. Take care that the "before and after" photos are not stock photos. Some dentists do use those, but it is easy to recognize those types of photos these days. Again, the bottom line is your comfort level with the person you choose to be your dentist.

WHAT A COSMETIC DENTIST CAN DO TO FIX YOUR SMILE

If I had to describe what a cosmetic dentist does, I would say that a cosmetic dentist makes your smile better. This encompasses anything that a dentist might do to enhance your smile: bonding, whitening, crowns, veneers, gum re-countering, etc. Almost any dental procedure that enhances your smile would fall into the area of cosmetic dentistry. For example, implants are an element of cosmetic dentistry. If you were missing a front tooth, an implant can be used to correct that problem. That is why cosmetic dentistry is not a specialty because so many things can be included in this category. Bonding was probably the first method of cosmetic dentistry. It was used to fill in and cosmetically enhance the teeth. For example, if a child fell off a bicycle and chipped his permanent tooth, bonding was used to fill in the chip. If an adult had an accident and knocked out half of his front tooth, bonding material would be used to build up the tooth and fill in the missing section. Bonding is a composite filler mixture of resin and glass that mimics the appearance and the strength of a tooth. Dentists can use it to repair a chipped, cracked, or broken tooth so that it appears as it did before. The bonding material is placed on the front of the tooth, polished, and then hardened with a curing light. Bonding can fill in cavities or gaps between the teeth, and is also a very good way to change the size, shape, and position of the teeth. Bonding is much less expensive and faster than the orthodontic treatment or veneers.

Of course, there is also a negative side. Bonding stains over the years. Since bondings are porous instead of porcelain, they absorb color. Around five to seven years after any bonding treatment, it will be time to change the bondings (because they will start to change color) or replace the bondings with porcelain to avoid that future problem. Some patients may not be able to afford the cost of veneers so they initially choose bondings. Several years later, when they are in a better financial position, they can afford to replace the bondings with veneers. This may also be the case with a young person, who should not have veneers done because the mouth is still changing. Dentists use bonding as a way to correct the immediate problem. Later in life, the young person can choose to replace the bondings with veneers.

In some cases, veneers may be the best option from the beginning. Veneers last between 10 and 15 years and cover the entire outer portion of the tooth. Veneers are very thin lens like porcelain pieces that cover the teeth in order to change their shape, size, and color according to a patient's need and preference. The dentist must first prepare the tooth by removing 0.5 to 1 millimeter of the enamel. Next, the dentist will make an impression of the teeth and send it to a laboratory. The laboratory makes the veneers based on the impressions, returns the veneers to the dentist's office, and the dentist places them on the patient's teeth. Since the laboratory can take up to two weeks to return the finished veneers, dentists place a temporary material over the tooth so that the patient does not need to worry about showing contoured teeth while the veneers are being made.

When a patient comes into our dental office, we make sure that we can meet the patient's expectations by finding out what the patient is asking for—and why. Again, the dentist needs to understand his or her patient and the patient needs to feel confident that the dentist is listening and understands the request. Ultimately, the dentist must be able to deliver the patient's request. Sometimes, a patient's expectations may be too high. In that case, the dentist has to let the patient know that the outcome may not exactly be what they are looking for. Communication between the dentist and patient is probably one of the most important elements in cosmetic dentistry.

Many patients come into my office because they are embarrassed by their smile or do not like their smile for some reason. Maybe they have cracks, gaps between the teeth, chips, or discolored teeth. Maybe they think that their teeth are too small or they show a large area of their gums when they smile. They could even be missing a tooth and don't want to smile out of embarrassment. It just depends on the person and what he or she wants to achieve by enhancing his or her smile.

WHO IS A CANDIDATE FOR COSMETIC DENTISTRY

Traditionally, most cosmetic dentistry patients were females over 40 years old, searching for a way to enhance their appearance by changing their smiles. Now, I would say that dentists see just as many male patients who want to enhance their smiles as female patients, along with younger patients. For example, a young patient came into my office requesting porcelain veneers. I tried to explain that she has time to do this later, but that other available options would not be as invasive or permanent. Even though it's now possible to place "no prep veneers" on top of the tooth without shaving the enamel (these are removable), the problem is that this procedure requires the perfect candidate and most patients are not a candidate. Using veneers on such a young patient commits her to a lifetime of veneers, since she will likely have to replace them every 10 to 15 years.

I explained this to my young patient, and I also explained some of the other methods that could enhance her smile besides veneers. We did some enamel re-contouring, reshaping some of the teeth a little bit, and the results were amazing. We also whitened her teeth. These methods are still considered cosmetic dentistry, even though they are not invasive or complicated. The result was a tremendous enhancement of the patient's smile. She could not believe that we accomplished it with just minor alterations.

One of my other patients was a young woman who had survived an automobile accident but was in terrible shape with missing and cracked teeth. She was in tears when she came to my office. In addition to the emotional and physical trauma of the automobile accident, she also had the trauma caused by her smile. Though her lip had healed from the cuts, her teeth were not as easy to repair. Most of the damage was done to the top teeth. We replaced the missing teeth with implants and then placed ten veneers on her top teeth to cover the cracks and broken teeth. We also whitened the top and bottom teeth. Even when we put on the temporaries, she was amazed and in tears because she could smile with confidence, without seeing her ruined smile.

A few months later, she met her future husband; both of them are still my patients. She says that she met her husband because we changed her smile. While I am not convinced that this was the case, I am quite sure that it gave her back her confidence. This is what people look for when they enhance their smile: confidence. People who smile are more approachable. If they do not like their smile, they often hide it. Cosmetic dentistry is life-changing. With it, some people who may have been perceived as grim or unhappy can smile and show the world their true nature and personality with confidence. Other people will see you as you see yourself. People see you differently when you smile, because you seem more confident and easier to approach.

For people who have old, unattractive fillings that steal their confidence, many aesthetic restorations can correct the problem. One method, called direct fillings, is created in the dentist's office while indirect options are processed in a lab. Direct fillings are a type of composite that the dentist will mix and use in-office to fill the tooth. Composite is much better than it was many years ago and looks much more realistic than silver fillings. These fillings last from five to ten years before beginning to absorb stains and change color. They are also prone to leakage as they age.

Indirect restorations are also available. One of the options is lab-processed composite, which is less porous than a direct restoration composite and therefore more stain-resistant. Other options include porcelain restorations, which are porcelain fillings (called inlays or outlays) in which the tooth, cavity, or old filling gets replaced. Porcelain restorations are made either in a laboratory or by E4D CAD/CAM machines. An impression is taken of the tooth, the laboratory makes the insert or replaces the part that's missing, and then the inlay/onlay is bonded into place. These types of fillings are much stronger and last longer than direct fillings. Porcelain is very close to enamel so this type of restoration does not stain like composite does. It looks just like a normal tooth and people cannot tell the difference between a real tooth and the porcelain one.

Movie stars and celebrities are frequent patients for cosmetic dentists because their livelihood depends on their smile and the way they look. However, more and more regular people want to look younger and more beautiful, and a beautiful smile (not a "denture smile") is associated with being young and healthy. Younger teeth tend to be a bit bigger and not yet ground down. However, as we age, our lips drop and cover more of our smile. We can appear younger by reversing that aging process with crowns, veneers, and reshaping.

Cosmetic dentistry is the way stars get that great-looking smile and keep it as they age. They use cosmetic dentistry such as crowns, veneers, reshaping, and whitening. Sometimes, they even use products such as Invisalign® to correct their smiles, like Tom Cruise did. One of his teeth was out of alignment with his face, so he had to have it shifted over. By simply asking their dentist, patients can have the same things done as the stars do. Cosmetic procedures do not need to be major or drastic to make a difference. Even minor changes can make our smiles look much better. As they say, "Beauty is in the eye of the beholder." That is why it is so important to talk to your dentist about your expectations, so the dentist understands what you are asking for and what you expect.

My best advice to patients: be certain that you understand what you want and don't let anyone talk you into something you are not sure of. Sometimes the dentist makes a suggestion and the patient just follows it. However, since the patient is the one that has to wear that smile, he/she should be happy with the final outcome. For the most part, these procedures are not reversible. Once the cosmetic dental work is done, it is done. You can ask for advice but the final decision should be yours.

Of course, dentists want to help make your smile beautiful. However, we also want you to understand that your smile should be healthy. Visit your dentist for regular check-ups and cleanings in order to make sure that your mouth is free of any cavities or gum disease. We can build a beautiful house but you must have the proper foundation underneath, otherwise, it is not going to hold—it will all come crumbling down. Of course, a good dentist will check your gums and teeth to make sure that they are healthy and that your teeth are strong enough to withstand a mouth makeover that will last for years.

(This content should be used for informational purposes only. It does not create a doctor-patient relationship with any reader and should not be construed as medical advice. If you need medical advice, please contact a doctor in your community who can assess the specifics of your situation.)

4

INVESTMENT
IN YOURSELF

by Jack D. Griffin, Jr., D.M.D.

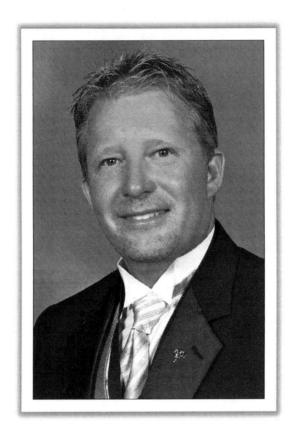

Jack D. Griffin, Jr., D.M.D.
Eureka Smile Center
Eureka, Missouri
www.eurekasmile.com

Dr. Jack D. Griffin has an exceptional practice in St Louis county Missouri where he and his staff perform all phases of general dentistry from high-end cosmetic procedures to "every day" restorative and preventive care.

Dr. Griffin is one of the most honored and awarded dentists in the country. He is one of a very few number of dentists to be awarded by his peers Diplomat status with the American Board of Aesthetic Dentistry (ABAD), accreditation with the American Academy of Cosmetic Dentistry (AACD) and Mastership in the Academy of General Dentistry (AGD). Due to his experience and knowledge, Dr. Griffin teaches and lectures about the various aspects and techniques of cosmetic dentistry. He also meets with other dentists to help them learn about practice management, digital photography, direct bonding techniques, cosmetic veneers, and CAD/CAM dentistry.

Dr. Griffin has taken over 2000 hours of continuing education since graduating dental school... his commitment to keep learning keeps him at the top of his profession. Being at the top of his profession, he is often asked write articles for prestigious professional journals such as Practical Procedures and Aesthetic Dentistry, Journal of Oral Health, Canadian Journal of Restorative Dentistry and Prosthodontics, Compendium, Dentistry Today, Inside Dentistry, Dental Economics, and Contemporary Esthetics, Dental Products Report and Dental Equipment and Materials.

INVESTMENT IN YOURSELF

Is your smile getting better or worse with time? Your smile is one of the first things people notice about you. If you can answer "yes" to any of these questions, it may be time to consider a smile enhancement.

- When you see photos of yourself, do your teeth, lips, and mouth look as good as they should?

- Do you feel self-conscious about your smile when you look in the mirror?

- Does it seem that others stare at your less-than-perfect pearly whites?

- Are your teeth becoming darker, more yellow, less straight, shorter, or more aged than they used to be?

Next, these three things need to be decided: how, what, and where. First, identify the characteristics that you don't like about your smile and what qualities you like in a great smile. There are many treatment options, from a very conservative treatment with minimal expense, to more complex treatments requiring more of an investment. Knowing a bit about dental cosmetic options before starting can make decisions easier and take away some of the apprehension associated with such an important aesthetic decision.

Everything makes a cosmetic difference, from choosing the right team to the right procedures. Obtaining a fantastic smile is not as hard as you may think, as long as you can identify your aesthetic needs, make an educated treatment decision, and correctly choose the office to do the procedures. Once these criteria are satisfied, a smile enhancement may be the absolute best investment you can ever make in yourself.

WHOM DO I CHOOSE?

The first choice to make is where to have the treatment done. The goal is to find an experienced team of knowledgeable staff members who listen to your desires and thoroughly explain comprehensive aesthetic treatment options. This decision can be difficult for any patient and takes some due diligence and a little research. It's more than just asking friends or relatives for a recommendation and might be more than having it done at the family dentist.

Don't be thrown off by the alphabet soup of letters after a doctor's name, and don't allow memberships to sway you too much. Instead, pay attention to achievements, honors, and certificates of advanced training. Since there is no recognized "specialist" in dental aesthetics, anyone with a dental license can make aesthetic changes. However, working with a doctor who has earned recognized accomplishments in the field can give you peace of mind.

Memberships generally indicate that a doctor has paid dues to belong to an organization. Usually, professionals can join without needing to display any qualification, test, or ex-perience. Memberships in various organizations are not a bad thing by any means. In fact, the membership may imply a special interest or level of commitment by that doctor towards a special field of care such as cosmetic dentistry. Memberships in these organizations are critical for staff training, technique advancements, and research. However, some memberships may indicate nothing more about a doctor than his ability to keep current on dues.

Many areas of dentistry offer advancement. In other words, doctors seeking more expertise and enhanced group status in certain areas can engage in testing, case presentations, advanced study, and peer review. Aesthetic dental associations like the American Academy of Cosmetic Dentistry (AACD), American Board of Aesthetic Dentistry (ABAD), and the American

Society of Dental Aesthetics (ASDA) offer advancement to dentists through three means: real patient cases, evaluations for cosmetic excellence, and commitment to the discipline. There's no guarantee of a great result, but all things being equal, these awards may separate one doctor from another and give you confidence in your choice.

WEBSITE AND GALLERY

Internet usage is a primary source of patient research and education. Valuable online information may lead to choosing a great office, learning about specific procedures, and even social media rankings. A well-designed, professional website may establish your first contact with an office; its layout, organization, and style may reflect the dental office and staff. Look for the doctor's credentials, any emphasis on aesthetic procedures, and photographs of actual patients.

The gallery is possibly the most important feature of any cosmetic dental website. Detailed photographs of in-office aesthetic treatment may be the best way of comparing one doctor to another, in terms of cosmetic excellence. Great photos with dramatic smile enhancements, using a variety of techniques, can be an important way to see improvements made by dental staff and can go a long way in calming your fears about a doctor.

Most aesthetically-oriented offices develop a portfolio of actual patient cases, showing photographs on the walls, in-office portfolio books, or on a website gallery. It's very important that the patient sees smile enhancements done by that particular staff to see the look, style, and harmony with the face. Essentially, it should show work that you wouldn't mind being done on yourself. Viewing these images is an important step in building your confidence in the doctor and staff and may be some means of choosing one staff over another.

Notice the full-face smiles for the facial development, close-up photos showing realistic contours, and teeth that are not all one color. Teeth should look bright and youthful with character and natural contours. Many galleries are filled with young women with very white teeth which may not look very natural or realistic. Remember that the patient probably chose her own final color.

Before or during treatment, we recommend that a patient go to our office or website gallery to choose a case or two that particularly impressed him or her. This helps establish a beginning idea of color, size, and anatomy of teeth that is pleasing to the patient. These "before and after" images can help you narrow down the characteristics that you like to help you relax about your own smile improvements.

The staff of the dentist is critical to your treatment experience. We call our staff "the waking gallery". Most of them have experienced the very treatments that we do daily on the patients, so they have confidence in the dentist after having seen firsthand what can be done. The staff has often had their teeth enhanced as well, which gives them an understanding of treatment and experiences that they share with the patients. Nothing can replace a patient talking directly to someone wearing veneers, orthodontically straightened teeth, or bleached teeth.

"WHAT CAN WE DO FOR YOU?"

It's very difficult when a female patient brings in a photo of Halle Berry and says, "I want to look like that." That desired change may be a bit more than the staff can deliver, just like making all men look like Channing Tatum would be nice but unrealistic. It must be understood that we are enhancing your smile, to make you a better you, and not giving you someone else's smile.

The ultimate goal in any dental treatment is a happy patient. First, and most importantly, the staff must listen to the patient. ("What can we do for you?") Often, patients have a basic idea of wanting whiter, straighter, and more youthful teeth but aren't exactly sure of what treatment are really asking for. The dental staff helps identify specific patient desires and then tempers those expectations within the limitations of oral tissues, dental materials, and the patient's foundation. You must be confident that the dental team is really listening and that we involve you in treatment discussion and decision-making process. This will help calm ever-present apprehensions that appear when considerable aesthetic therapy is being done.

I am very fortunate in teaching aesthetic dentistry techniques to many doctors across the country and hear constantly that the ultimate frustration is also the elusive goal of every conscientious practitioner: "What does the patient really want?" How do we get them to put into words the vision they have for themselves so that neither patient nor doctor is frustrated in the end? Often patients aren't sure what they are really asking for.

Look in the mirror closely to see what you don't like. Is it color, size, space, crowding, narrow jaws, protruding teeth, missing teeth, gummy smile, or a combination of several things you don't like? You are the one who owns your smile, and it's important to share all of your concerns with the dental team so they can meet your treatment expectations. Look at smiles that you really like and try to identify their pleasing traits. Not just the natural beauty of that particular person, celebrity, or model but what you like specifically about the teeth or smile.

PHOTOS DON'T LIE

Photography can be an indispensable ally. In our office at the initial consultation, we put smile and close-up photos of the patient on a TV monitor and ask the patient a very simple question: "What don't you like about your smile?" This gives us a great starting point in formulating a cosmetic plan by having the patient identify specific problems, which is much more helpful to the staff than just saying, "I don't like my smile." From here we consider tissue health, function of the mouth, and the materials needed to achieve these corrections.

The staff must cultivate a trust with the patient by combining active listening with the assurance that comes with aids such as smile simulations, model "wax ups" of proposed treatment, and a thorough explanation of treatment options. Then we can plan correctly, communicating realistic expectations to the patient.

We consistently make dramatic, patient-centered improvements, but perfection only comes when the patient is very pleased with the outcome. Be careful when using extreme wording like "perfect" or "exactly like". While we have a high level of confidence in what we can deliver, we want to be realistic so that we don't have disappointment later. The more information that the dental staff can gather from the patient makes it more likely that a patient will be well pleased after treatment.

SIMULATIONS

Many offices offer computer simulations. A photo is taken, put into computer software, and teeth are copied from a library and placed onto the patient photo. While these approximate simulations can help the patient see what they would look like with teeth enhancement, they are very often impossible to clinically duplicate because they don't take into account the confines of real oral tissue response. Computer simulations do not account for soft tissue changes such as lip position, realistic gum placement, or facial response to contours. Therefore, patients must be warned that their hopes can be falsely elevated by software changes. Maintain realistic expectations and shoot for drastic improvements on "a better you" rather than perfection with your smile.

THE FACE

Now that you've chosen a team of staff wisely and have an idea of what you don't like about your smile, understand that cosmetic dentistry includes much more than straighter, whiter teeth. Balancing the character and position of the teeth with the muscles and tissues of the face is what makes a great smile. When careful aesthetic enhancement of these structures is done within the realm of realistic patient desires, a gain in beauty can be appreciated.

The true goal of aesthetic dentistry today is to provide enhancements that look and function naturally while meeting patient expectations. It is as much about the lower face as it is about tooth position, color, and shape. The placement, size, and volume of the teeth affect the facial support muscles and how the skin and other tissues hang over them. Dental structure is the major determinant of the appearance of the lower face. Improperly positioned teeth with a lack of oral volume can cause a collapsed look with sunken cheeks, unsupported lips, wrinkling, and an aged appearance.

Conversely, large bulky teeth that are flared out or too far forward can make the patient strain to close and make the lips too far forward and full. The desire for whiter, straighter teeth must be meet with respect to facial harmony and the physiology of chewing. The guidance of an experienced, well-trained dental team (matched with your realistic expectations) is critical to long-term success.

VENEERS: PLASTIC OR PORCELAIN

Decades ago, the current dental aesthetic restorative revolution began with the advent of veneering materials. Their use in dentistry cannot be under-emphasized because of the dramatic "overnight" improvements seen in just one or two treatment appointments. Veneers are ultra-thin coverings that are placed on the tooth surface to correct many patient-displeasing traits such as spaces, color, and alignment. They are extended only from the front of the tooth to cover any defects.

Two major materials are used in dental veneers today: composite and porcelain. Composite materials are a resin (plastic) with glass particles and are today's choice for tooth-colored fillings. (Remember that just replacing silver fillings or correcting decay can provide a significant cosmetic improvement in some cases.) In a process widely known as "bonding", the composite material is placed directly onto a prepared tooth. It is a wonderful aesthetic material for small space closure, tooth chipping, and even minor position correcting. This material is placed by the doctor, sculpted, and finished in the mouth—often within one appointment.

However, composite may not the best material for durability and is not the first choice as a veneering material. It tends to chip, stain, and break much more often than porcelain. Patients can expect maintenance issues over time when composite is used to correct more than the smallest of defects. Composite use in veneer cases has decreased greatly with time because of the advent of other materials like ceramics.

The ultimate aesthetic material is porcelain, a type of ceramic. It's used as the predominant smile makeover material because of its high level of aesthetics, resistance to wear, diversity, and durability. This material is stronger than composite and therefore can be made thinner, about the thickness of a fingernail, with an amazing ability to enhance the smile. The cosmetic world was changed forever when porcelain was first used for veneers; it was, and still is, the best cosmetic combination of strength and beauty.

The range of smile detractors that can be corrected with the porcelain restoration is almost limitless. Dark teeth can be masked and turned into any color the patient wants, short worn teeth restored to normal lengths, spaces closed, and misaligned teeth straightened. There is no discoloration with time and repairs are seldom needed. It's truly an amazing material.

Newer porcelain or ceramic materials provide an even higher level of aesthetics and strength. Full tooth coverings (crowns) and tooth replacements (bridges) can be done without metal, which eliminates the darkening at the gum line seen around metal-based crowns topped with porcelain.

Porcelain veneers are more of an initial investment than composite, but the benefits make the additional cost of investment worth it in many cases. These materials are truly an aesthetic wonder and are often the standard in almost any comprehensive aesthetic rehabilitation.

MINIMAL GRINDING

Conservative treatment is the current mantra of dental aesthetics. Newer materials provide such a high level of beauty and strength that, in many cases, very minimal tooth preparation is needed—if at all. "Dr. Griffin only reduces the minimum amount of tooth structure that will ensure an excellent result," we assure our patients. Both patients and dentists prefer that grinding be minimized or avoided as long as an excellent cosmetic outcome can be obtained and there are no thick teeth that stick out. In the absence of decay or disease, conservation of natural tooth structure is always wise whenever possible. Also, we preserve the natural tooth structure by lessening or eliminating grinding on the teeth, leading to stronger restorations with less chance of future clinical problems or sensitivity. Our desire is to provide an improved, long-lasting smile that needs little future repair or maintenance.

If you have decay, old restorations, or bulky teeth, more tooth preparation must be done to meet the long-term needs of your bite and the cosmetic goals of treatment.

With paper-thin porcelain or composite bonded to the outer surface of the teeth, great cosmetic enhancements can be done with minimal tooth preparation. Depending upon the condition and position of the teeth, a very slight roughening of the enamel surface is all that is often needed for an excellent cosmetic result and long-lasting beauty.

THE NUMBER

In almost every cosmetic consultation regarding veneers, the patient asks, "How many teeth do we treat?" We always reply, "It depends." If the desire is to significantly change color on only the front four or six teeth, the smile would look like two distinctly different colors and show everyone else that you had something done. Also, any significant changes to tooth shape and size will show when you smile.

Since most people show a minimum of the top eight to ten teeth in a full smile, that is a starting point when talking about porcelain veneer smile makeovers. In less drastic cases, just correcting one or two teeth can make a dramatic difference. Closure of a space between the front two teeth, replacing stained restorations, repairing a chip—porcelain or composite—can be done on a few teeth if the overall color of the teeth remains unchanged.

Plans almost always differ from patient to patient, due to unique circumstances and needs, provided that the patient's desires are met without regrets. We have never heard a patient regret treating too many teeth but have often heard, "I wish I would have done more." When making an investment in your smile, a compromise in treatment may be a poorer return on your investment than a plan that may cost more in the beginning.

REPLACE THEM

If you are missing teeth, the cheeks and muscles of the face always sink in to some degree. When teeth are missing, the bones shrink (resorption) over time so that missing teeth cause loss of both tooth and bone volume. The roots of your teeth stimulate the maintenance of bone that supports your lower face. Therefore, replacing teeth not only provides more chewing force, but also provides the stimulation to keep tissues from sinking, collapsing, and some wrinkling around the mouth.

Implants have completely changed the way missing teeth are replaced. Implants are root-shaped titanium pieces that are placed in the position of the original tooth root. As long as there is enough ridge or bone in the area of the lost tooth, the patient goes through a minimal surgical technique and a healing period (osseointegration), and a tooth is placed onto the implant. It's possible to achieve excellent aesthetics, great function, and replacement of tooth volume to reduce the collapse of facial tissues without grinding on neighboring teeth.

Implants can create a high level of aesthetics when replacing missing front teeth. The success rate for implants is more than 95% for ten years. Again, with the facial structure as the primary goal, placing an implant not only replaces the tooth but also stimulates the bone of the jaw to remain in place without age-related shrinking. Without tooth roots or implants, both the jaw and supports for lips and facial soft tissues will become smaller.

Currently used materials for cemented, conventional bridges require far less reduction than in years past, without the use of metal. Some preparation of the adjacent teeth must be done to provide the proper clearance for bridge materials and to ensure proper placement. Tooth replacement, in the form of cemented bridges or implants, is one of the most important factors in lower facial cosmetics and preservation of a youthful amount of structural bone.

MOVE THEM

Orthodontic treatment is probably the most conservative and oldest cosmetic treatment of all. It should be considered in cases that involve improperly positioned teeth, rotated teeth, crowding, spacing, bite issues, and general tooth alignment. Moving teeth today is much different than in previous years. Braces have changed considerably with the use of tooth-colored brackets, more comfortable wires, and faster treatment. Tooth-colored brackets are often used on adults and are not nearly as visible as old-fashioned metal brackets.

Aligners like Invisalign® can also make dramatic smile improvements without using brackets or wires. These clear, thin, digitally-made, retainer-like trays make small, continuous tooth movements. The patient wears the aligners 24/7 except when eating or brushing teeth. As long as the patient wears them and the fit is good, they certainly move teeth if used in the right cases. In some cases, they don't have the same precise movement or bite-correcting capabilities as with traditional tooth-colored braces, but they can correct many smile defects if the teeth are free of decay and restoration.

Orthodontics offers patients the ability to have an awesome smile without the need for dental restorations. However, the tradeoff is a time commitment of months to years, depending on the alignment issues and the amount of necessary tooth movement. Teeth continue to move after orthodontic treatment, so a commitment to retainer use after tooth movement ensures that teeth stay in the desired location.

BLEACH THEM

Particularly when teeth are in a good alignment, bleaching can make dramatic improvements. Bleaching is a very safe way to remove stains within the tooth itself by breaking down the attachment between staining materials and the tooth, which results in whiter teeth. Fillings, older dental work, decay, enamel defects, and other issues may have to be dealt with before or after bleaching to gain the maximum cosmetic benefit.

Since whitening kits are sold at Wal-Mart, Walgreens, and CVS, why have it done in a professional office? First of all, the bleaching material is probably as inexpensive in the dental office as in the grocery store but far more effective. Most offices provide special custom-made trays for each patient, ensuring the proper contact of bleach with the teeth. This allows for a conservation of bleach gel—only a very small amount is needed with each application. Most offices recommend that bleach be applied all night long or one to two times per day for 30–45 minutes each time.

There are a variety of bleach types and strengths with different combinations of desensitizers and bleaching power. The dental staff determines the proper material, the type of bleach, and any sensitivity-reduction protocol. Several gels can be used inside the bleaching trays to reduce or eliminate any unwelcome sensations that occur when some patients whiten their teeth. By alternating nights with bleach and desensitizing gels, even the most sensitive patients can get whiter teeth.

Professional guidance is important to monitor effectiveness and tissue responses to the material.

In-office bleaching can accelerate the bleaching process but may not improve the final outcome—just the speed of the result. Even the faster systems (using high-powered bleach along with light exposure) require some at-home bleaching with trays to maintain the new color. Even some difficult tooth staining, such as dark gray or brown teeth with "banding", can be lightened with methodical, consistent bleaching. If tooth position, shape, and length are all sound, bleaching may be the best "bang for the buck" of any cosmetic procedure.

GUM TREATMENT

One overlooked aspect of aesthetic therapy is the shape and position of the gums (gingiva). When an excessive amount of gum tissue shows during a smile, it takes away from the whiteness of the teeth and overall pleasantness of the face. Often minor reshaping can be done with a laser, which can make a drastic improvement in treatment. Laser reshaping can provide a better environment for cleaning, plaque control, and overall gum health while improving cosmetics. Laser therapy has become a staple in cosmetic dentistry, making gum tissue less noticeable when smiling and balancing tissues to improve smile proportions.

Occasionally, with certain defects, gingival plastic surgery can be done to enhance the look and health of the teeth. This may involve a specialist and can be used to make teeth appear longer, correct gum disease, or to decrease the amount of visible soft tissue. The gingival should not be overlooked in any cosmetic case. Commitment to long-term home and in-office cleanings cannot be under-emphasized for the preservation of your smile investment.

INVEST IN YOURSELF

A full cosmetic enhancement often involves more than one of the techniques mentioned. For instance, it is very popular for patients to have porcelain veneers on the upper teeth while only doing bleaching or orthodontics on the less visible lowers. Often, the patient only needs composite bonding to close a space or just tooth replacement and color changes. The key for the staff is to find what the patient wants, reassure them, make a thorough plan, and deliver great work.

Fees vary greatly by procedure, office, and location. Porcelain restorations are at the top end of the investment scale since they involve the most artistry, technique, and staff ability. They also correct the most imperfections at once. The trade-off for this larger investment is that the change is almost instant, the results are relatively maintenance-free, and patient discomfort is minimal.

Orthodontics may be less money than several porcelain veneers, but the tradeoff is the associated time and discomfort. Bleaching is on the other end of the investment scale: it's relatively inexpensive but can only affect color—not tooth position, lip support, or other cosmetic considerations.

Cosmetic dentistry is the most rewarding part of dental practice because of the incredible gratitude that we receive from patients after treatment. We work diligently to match the proper aesthetic treatment with the facial tissues, biting physiology, and patient desires. When all of these steps come together, the excellence achieved can be life changing as our patients' self-confidence is greatly increased.

(This content should be used for informational purposes only. It does not create a doctor-patient relationship with any reader and should not be construed as medical advice. If you need medical advice, please contact a doctor in your community who can assess the specifics of your situation.)

5

THREE STEPS TO CHOOSING THE RIGHT COSMETIC DENTIST

by Tanya L. DeSanto, D.D.S.

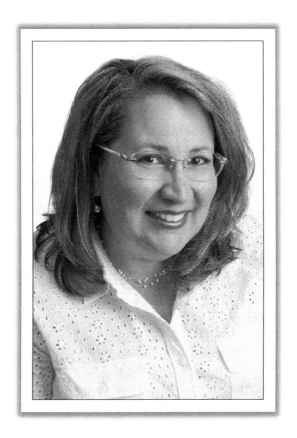

Tanya L. DeSanto, D.D.S.
Prairie Dental Group
Springfield, Illinois
www.prairiedentalgroup.com

Dr. Tanya L. DeSanto, a graduate of Northwestern University, has been creating beautiful smiles for adults and children for over 20 years. She is committed to providing her patients with exceptional state of the art cosmetic services giving them the beautiful smile they desire.

Dr. DeSanto was recently inducted into the International College of Dentists, the oldest and largest international honor society for dentists. She is a teacher and a leader in her community, Springfield, Illinois.

In addition to her long list of accomplishments, Dr. DeSanto is a sustaining member of the American Academy of Cosmetic Dentistry, a Past President of the G.V. Black District Dental Society, the Chicago Dental Society, the American Dental Association, American Association of Women Dentists, the Dental Organization for Conscious Sedation and a founding member of the Prairie Academy of Cosmetic Dentistry.

THREE STEPS TO CHOOSING THE RIGHT COSMETIC DENTIST

Having an attractive smile is important because it is the way that you greet the world. It is the highlight and focal point of your face. Your smile is your most notable feature, so it needs to be your best feature.

Choosing the right cosmetic dentist to bring out the best features of you smile is important if you want to achieve spectacular results. I would suggest that you take the following three steps to find the right cosmetic dentist, who can meet your goals and desires.

First, I recommend that you look at their education and training. It is exciting to be a dentist in today's modernized world because we have so many tools in our basket and research has come so far. As a cosmetic dentist, I am always searching for ways to improve my skills, techniques and abilities. I believe that by aspiring to achieve higher standards of education and training, a cosmetic dentist is able to produce artistic, high-quality results for each of their patients. One can never stop learning. One must surround themselves with all the world experts and organizations like the American Academy of Cosmetic Dentistry, the International College of Dentistry, where I received my fellowship.

The second step in finding the right cosmetic dentist is by looking at the dentist's gallery on the website. You can view anyone's gallery, of before and after pictures on their website. Cosmetic dentists are proud of their work, so look at the work they have done on other patients and see what you think. The photography demonstrates it all. I think it is interesting to see the life-changing effects of cosmetic dentistry on actual patients.

The third and most important step you should take when searching for a cosmetic dentist is to check referrals from other patients. Someone who has had a smile makeover and who is very happy with his or her smile is willing to talk to other people about the dentist and his or her experience with that dentist. I think that, of all the people that come to our practice, the number one way they arrive is through a referral from a previous patient. I think you cannot go wrong if you take all three steps when searching for a cosmetic dentist. You should feel right at home when you go into the office.

STATE-OF-THE-ART COSMETIC DENTISTRY AT AFFORDABLE PRICES

In our practice, distance does not seem to be a barrier for our patients. We are more of a regional dental office rather than simply local. Patients travel long distances for our services and we cater to that in our office. When people come in for a consultation, we review all of the things we can do for them and we set up two visits to accomplish their individual choices. Our lab is a very important team member in this process.

Our town is also part of the reason why distance is not a problem for patients utilizing our practice. Our town is the home of Abraham Lincoln, so there are many things to do and see while a patient is in town. We can schedule a patient's two appointments within the same week so that patients planning to stay the entire week can take in the sights. Some people come for the first appointment and then return to the office according to their schedule and their plans. It seems to work well for us and our patients, furthering the notion that distance is not a factor. Another advantage is that our area generally has lower prices compared to some of the larger cities.

Therefore, it is very affordable to have cosmetic procedures done at Prairie Dental Group. Our patients receive state-of-the-art dentistry at affordable prices. That is probably the driving factor for many people, as cosmetic dentistry is something that is not typically covered by dental insurance, causing most of the expense to come from out of pocket. This is a one-time investment and people are beginning to see the benefits of cosmetic dentistry.

IT TAKES A TEAM TO GET OUTSTANDING RESULTS

You also want to choose a dentist who uses a state-of-the-art laboratory. As a dentist, I believe that it is vital to choose a state-of-the-art laboratory to back you and your skills so that your results are outstanding. I personally feel I have the most amazing dental laboratory in the whole world. In fact, my master technician was just honored at our academy meeting last fall. I am really proud of him and he is definitely my right hand in creating exceptional results for my clients. I also believe that the materials a dentist uses and the dental staff are big factors when assessing the skill of a dentist. Most of my staff has been with me at least twenty years. Your staff is an important part of your entire team. It takes an excellent team to give outstanding results. When you have a team that works well together, patients are the true beneficiaries. Ultimately, this is what you want when you choose a cosmetic dentist as well—a dentist with exceptional skill and who has put together an amazing team.

When cosmetic dentistry is your passion, as it is mine, a part of having that fervor is being attracted to others that have that same excitement. When you have that passion, you will want to work with others who share that same passion, whether it is your staff, lab, or other dentists. When you are striving to work your way up in the academy, there are laboratories who are working their way up in the academy as well, and they have to submit cases just as we have to submit cases. That is actually how I met my lab technician: he was striving for his accreditation just as I was for my own. I believe that, when you want something and you endeavor to be your best at it, you fill your surroundings with people who are striving for the similar things. I believe all dentists have access to great labs. However, it is all about whether a dentist has the passion and takes the time to find an exceptional lab to partner with to provide exceptional services to his or her patients.

We have a magazine in Springfield that is one of those city magazines—a big, oversized, glossy publication. It's a wonderful way to show the public the artistic work that we do and how much we can accomplish through cosmetic dentistry. Each season I take one of our makeover patients and put them in the magazine in a large ad. It is usually a face everybody knows, and now it has become a trend to see who we publish in the magazine every issue. People like to see what changes we can make to a person's smile with cosmetic dentistry and it is exciting for our patients to be featured in the publication. Now when I finish with someone, he or she asks, "Am I going to be in the magazine?" Everybody wants to be in it. It has taken on a life of its own.

PEOPLE WANT TO KNOW, IS IT WORTH THE EFFORT?

When people ask me, "Is it worth the effort?" I tell them, "If you want to know if it is worth the effort, you need to talk to the people who have been there." I refer them to the magazine and tell them to pick up any issue and talk to one of those people in the magazine. Any of them will be happy to answer that question. Each one of them will tell you it has been the best thing he or she has ever done. I think that you should go to people who have been where you are right now. You should ask the people who, like me, have done the work, but that is only half of it. Then you should go to the other half: the people who have received the work. If you go to the people who received the work, you are going to get your answer. It is definitely worth it. You will hear many times that it was the best thing they ever did. Finding a cosmetic dentist who knows how to deliver, that is who you want to use for your cosmetic work.

You cannot overestimate the importance of a gorgeous smile. It makes a huge difference in the lives of patients. If I had to sum up what I love the most about my job, it is sharing the experience of how a great smile can change a person's life. When I have completed the cosmetic work for a patient, the number one comment I hear from him at the post-op visit is, "I wish I would have done this ten years ago." I hear that all the time. That is the exact comment and the number is ten every time. People love that I bring back the youthful smile they have lost over the years or I give them a smile that they have always wanted. I think this is one item on many people's bucket lists.

A great smile gives people confidence and improves the way they carry themselves. It gives them that boost to do more, laugh more and perform better on so many levels, whether it is a stay-at-home mom or the CEO of a big company. It is amazing to see what happens when a person has a smile that she loves. I cannot tell you the number of people that come back to me, maybe six months to a year later, and they look very different. One of my patients just opened up the biggest cross-fit gym in Springfield. It is almost as if I am feeding this transformation. It is so exciting because it is all positive. So many good things come from enhancing your smile. Not one person among all of those I have ever helped during my long career has regretted having cosmetic dentistry.

When you restore your smile, the result is a lifetime of confidence. I do not say that lightly because I have seen it and I continue to see it all the time. In each person that we help, I see how it changes that person's life. Restoring your smile is probably the best thing you could do for yourself for so many reasons: self-esteem, confidence, function, aesthetics, and more! Enhancing your smile is the easiest type of cosmetic procedure to obtain. If you want to do something to keep your youthful look, your smile is the easiest thing to tackle and the easiest thing to restore. Porcelain veneers can lighten up the 20 or 30 years worth of food, soda, coffee, and wine stains off your teeth.

Sometimes patients can do very small things to obtain a better smile, and we like to introduce these things to our patients. Some people have beautiful teeth but they might just be chipped and broken a bit from wear and tear. We can take care of these issues in the six-month check-up. If a tooth is chipped, uneven, or little rough, we will polish it and shape it during the check-up visit. There is no need to make a separate appointment. We try to keep things fine-tuned and maintained perfectly throughout the patient's dental life. It may be as simple as sculpting a tooth or changing angles to remove the appearance of wear and tear. We can bring back angles and curves with bonding that people have lost over the years from grinding and wear and tear. Not all changes need to involve multiple visits and greater costs.

THE PROCESS

For a smile makeover in my office, the first step is to make sure that the patient has healthy teeth and healthy gums. We do a thorough cleaning and take a full set of x-rays to determine if we have good bone and supporting structures to work with when evaluating a candidate for cosmetic dentistry. The public may not realize that some people are not a good candidates for cosmetic dentistry when they first come into my office. Sometimes we must work hard to get a patient into a situation where he or she becomes a good candidate for cosmetic procedures. If a person has gum disease, we have to treat that first before we can begin any other procedures. If there is any type of infection anywhere, we have to treat that first. Most of the time, people come in having have taken care of their teeth, and some simply want to enhance their smile rather than do a complete makeover. Sometimes it only takes a few small changes to accomplish the patient's goals.

In addition to ensuring that the patient's overall oral health makes him or her a good candidate for cosmetic work, the initial consultation is vital for the successful completion of the case. I have learned over the past few decades of practicing cosmetic dentistry that the success of any case is completely based on effective communication with the patient. You must find out what the patient is looking for and how you can meet and then exceed that patient's expectations. Understanding what the patient is looking for is the beginning point—this is the number one priority. If I am not sure that I completely understand what the patient wants, then we will take one extra step and whatever time it takes to ensure we are all on the same page. We will take models of the teeth and I will perform the work on these models to show the patient what he or she can expect before we do anything with the actual teeth. We go through many different procedures so that the patient can discover what he or she desires and so that my lab technician and I can fully understand that aspiration. Then we can talk about how we can achieve that for the patient.

When I consult with a patient, I want to give him or her, the perfect aesthetic look for his or her face and features. I look at what kind of things we need to change to accomplish that goal. Do we need to re-shape some teeth, reposition some teeth, change the color of the teeth or do all three of those things? What needs to change dictates what we are going to do or what our options are going to be for changing a person's smile. If I think the color looks really great but there are just a few teeth that are crooked, shifted, or just different, maybe clear aligners is the answer as opposed to other cosmetic treatments.

I first want to know is if a patient is satisfied with the color of his or her teeth. Sometimes people come into the office and want straight, white teeth. So they ask about products such as Invisalign® to straighten their teeth. If they do straighten their teeth to get them in the perfect position, are they going to love their teeth? The last thing I want to do is to straighten someone's teeth and then they are unhappy because they are not the color they had envisioned. When the patient wants super-white teeth, much lighter than I could ever do with bleaching, we opt for veneers to get the color that the patient desires. If that is the case, we do not need to do Invisalign® or clear aligners because veneers can change the position and color of the teeth. Again, it all goes back to good communication with the patient. Therefore, the first question I ask is, "Are you happy with the color of your teeth?" The answer to that question will give me an idea of what direction we need to go to meet the patient's goals.

People come to me because they want to love their smile. I am very, very particular about shade. That is probably my trigger. I am a little obsessed with shade, actually. I love a really fresh, natural smile.

The people that come to me are looking for help so they can love their smile. Sometimes that means that we need to address prior dental work that did not live up to their expectations or that they feel does not look pretty. When I see dental work that does not look good, I love to talk about options and what I can do for the patient to help them love their smile again.

It might be that they have old silver fillings in the mouth and they want to change to something that looks prettier. We can do that because silver fillings of the past were only mechanical plugs for the tooth. Now, with tooth-colored fillings, it is mechanical filling and a chemical bonding, so we can correct the problem with the tooth while giving the patient a pretty, natural look. Resin that we used 20 years ago tends to stain and they do not hold their surface color very well. They darken and become more of a yellow tone as they age, but now resins are just amazing. It is really exciting to talk to people about the new technology in the industry because they may not know. Perhaps the dentistry that they have in their mouth was the best available in those days. Now it is time to update, refresh, and modernize with the new technology. My job is to educate patients about options and guide them in a direction that will make them happy.

For teeth whitening, there are many alternatives. I think most people are not as interested in the over-the-counter whitening systems because they want results that they are unable to achieve at home—better results. Most people come to our office because they are ready for a dramatic change in the color of their teeth. We have several options for whitening teeth. My favorite is probably Zoom!®. I love it! I think I get the best results from that product. I have seen patients go eight shades whiter in my office using the Zoom!® product. I love knowing that, when I tell a patient I believe we can take them to this color, I will be really close to that (if not spot on) because of my experience in doing so many cases. I like having those very predictable results for people. There is also a new whitening system called Sinsational Smiles®. It has just been released and we have been using it in our office this year. It only takes about 20 minutes, so the process does not take as long as other whitening systems. We like it because a patient can lighten their teeth while getting numb for a filling. That way we can choose a lighter color for the filling.

There are over-the-counter toothpaste or whitening systems that you buy at the drug store. For some people, they may be only looking for a couple of shades of whitening and an over-the-counter product will let them achieve their modest objective. I think any amount of lightening is good and some people are very satisfied with their over-the-counter products. If a person is just looking for a little change in color, at-home products are safe, easy to use, and provide that little jump in color. For a younger patient who wants to whiten his or her teeth, such as a student going to the prom or a high school graduate, I tell the parents, "This is a perfect case for Crest White Strips®." These young kids do not have the stains that adults develop as we age. A white strip is probably all a young person needs to get what they think is whitening. For the rest of us, I don't think that is enough.

For most people, I think you need to whiten your teeth professionally with the 25% hydrogen peroxide active ingredient that is light-activated. I see the positive results every day. The easiest one hour you can spend on your teeth — the most bang for your buck, if you will — is whitening your teeth. If someone wants to change the dental fillings in the front, you want to whiten the teeth as much as you can to get the color as white as possible before you change the fillings. You can then pick the new filling color to match the new color of the teeth after whitening. You want to go as white as you can, so you should pick the whitest color possible to use, whether it is porcelain or bonding.

If you are going to do porcelain veneers, you do not need to lighten the teeth. The porcelain veneers that we put on your teeth are going to remain the same color for the rest of your life. If we only need to place a veneer on one of your teeth, we still must choose the color you want to have forever because the veneer color that we choose for today is going to be the color of your teeth for the rest of your life. In this case, we would do the Zoom!® whitening to get the teeth as white as possible and then match the veneer to the new tooth color. Now, the teeth all around the veneer will darken as you age, so it does force you to keep your teeth whiter. You have to use whitening trays every so often to keep your tooth color lighter; otherwise, you will have one white veneer and all the other teeth around that tooth will be a darker shade.

With the first Zoom!® whitening machine, some sensitivity was reported. I did not experience that, but I have heard of those cases. The new Zoom!® whitening machine, which really is not "new" anymore, still has some cases where sensitivity is an issue. Again, I have not experienced that issue with any of my patients. We do many of these procedures each week and, every once in a while, someone might have a tiny bit of sensitivity during the last session (there are three sessions to Zoom!® whitening) within the same one hour appointment. Sometimes, during the last session, people notice a little bit of sensitivity, but that is rare. I do not see the issue of sensitivity very often. The Zoom!® whitening system includes touch up trays that the patient takes home. Once in a while, I will need to give anti-sensitivity gel to a patient to use in the whitening tray at home to address the issue of sensitivity, if it arises on a rare occasion.

Teeth whitening is something just about anybody can do if he or she is a candidate for it. I recommend it to many people because it is very affordable and it is very easy and quick but makes a huge difference in appearance. I have done it myself and so has my family. We have even done bridal parties in our office where we use Zoom!® for the entire bridal party. Teeth whitening is just one of the many ways that we help our patients achieve the smile that they desire for those big days and the everyday.

Often, our teeth wear off from grinding so much over our lifespan, you see it especially in elderly patients. If we are going to bring back the shape of the teeth, we need to do much more than just whiten them. We have several options available to us to repair the damage that occurs with time. For younger people, who do not have a lot of wear and tear but may have teeth that are a bit crooked or maybe gaps in between the teeth, we can do a little bonding to repair the damage. If they like the color and shape of their teeth, you can add a little bonding and get very close to the look they desire. Everyone's needs are individualized. However, there is a very logical way to accomplish each person's goals. I think, through years of experience, I can educate patients about cosmetic dentistry and present patients with different ideas to meet their personal goals, and exceed them!

Not everything is as expensive as implants, veneers, or crowns. Just taking out two colored fillings that are stained or two old silver fillings that do not look good anymore will make a huge difference. I do not want people to think that the only thing we can do to restore their smile involves big, huge makeovers. Not everyone needs a gigantic change. Some people look so much better just lightening their teeth because they have beautiful teeth just the way they are, but they need to be whitened to brighten their smile. People may come into the office for a veneer consultation, but I do not always end up doing veneers for them. There are so many other things we can do to accomplish their goals. Some people assume that cosmetic dentists just bleach teeth and do veneers and that is all that we do. That is simply not the case.

Porcelain veneers have given us the option of changing the shape and position of a tooth while also correcting the color of the tooth. If we are doing porcelain veneers, that will require two very easy visits. The first visit is to perform prep work, to get the teeth in a position where we can place the veneers and to take impressions to fabricate the veneers. The impressions are sent to the laboratory for specific and detailed fabrication. At the second visit, we are ready to bond the porcelain veneers on the teeth.

Therefore, with the consultation included, that would be three visits to do everything. I feel it is very obtainable because we do it all the time. It works and people love it. A common question I often hear is, "How long is all of this going to last?" In my opinion, the veneers will last as long as you take care of them. If you maintain regular cleanings and dental check-ups, brush, and floss, there is no reason the veneers will look any different 10 or 20 years from the day we put them on your teeth. I can look at some of the cases I did 20 years ago and they still look great! Porcelain is so much more advanced and so beautiful in now versus how it looked in 1993. It makes me want to redo the veneers just to give the patient the newest look. Our dental materials are just so amazing today.

I firmly believe that CAD/CAM technology allows dentists to be more effective. Having a Cerec machine that creates perfect crowns with precise form fit and function in our office, allowing to deliver high tech care to our patients in a manner where we can control the process, to completion in minutes. For a patient who needs a crown, it allows us to complete the procedure in one visit, therefore avoiding the need for a patient to take time from work to come back for a second visit. Cerec technology is a good example of how far dentistry has come in recent years.

WHAT ARE THE OPTIONS FOR MISSING TEETH?

When you are looking at correcting missing teeth, we have several good options. Missing teeth affect more of our elderly population and you see these patients wearing dentures. That was definitely my grandparents' generation. Dentists often did not fix their teeth, so they pulled all of the teeth and gave them dentures. Unfortunately, many of those patients have worn dentures a very long time. This means they have lost a lot of their bone through aging and attrition and so the dentures do not stay in place very well anymore. What has really been rewarding in the last decade in our profession is the evolution of implants and mini-implants. People who are missing all of their teeth may be great candidates for either of these options.

Mini-implants are something new in our field, and they are very affordable. They are very small implants placed so that the dentures can be snapped into position. We can do mini-implants in just one day. We love doing this procedure because patients can walk out of our office with teeth that they can snap into their denture. Within one hour, we can make a new denture and lock these dentures in the patient's mouth. How great is that? If a patient has a denture that still looks good but it is just not fitting very well, we can use these mini-implants with the existing denture to correct the fit. It is an easy, affordable option for denture patients.

This leads me to talk about people that are missing one or two teeth. Full implants are a wonderful option and we do them all the time. They are just like having your own teeth again and there is nothing better than having your own teeth. People who are missing one or two teeth have several choices. If all of the other teeth are healthy, you want to make sure that the missing teeth are replaced as quickly as possible because there is the risk of drifting and it can alter your bite and cause wear on the opposite side. One option is to do a bridge, where we put a porcelain crown on both sides of the missing tooth and insert a porcelain crown in the middle that attaches to the crowns on each side. That procedure is just two quick visits and it works.

My favorite option however, would be to go with an implant that is exactly like your own tooth, yet stronger. A titanium implant is inserted into the bone, which sounds a little bit scary but it is safe and easy. It is probably easier than doing a filling, if you can believe that. After the implant is placed into the bone, we must wait four months before completing the process. This waiting period is called "osseointegration" because we are waiting for the titanium to fuse to your bone. Once that occurs, the cosmetic dentist makes a porcelain implant crown that goes on top of the implant. The implant is there and it is going to withstand anything. It will outlast all of your other, natural teeth. Implants are probably the most successful medical procedure a person can have done. They are 98% successful and nothing else in the field of dentistry or medicine is that successful. Implants are a very good investment as they restore your teeth and smile back to full function.

Another reason an implant is my first choice over a bridge is that you do not need to work with the adjacent teeth on either side of the missing space. You do not need to remove enamel from the other two teeth at all, in fact. A bridge is a great choice if you already have two crowns you are going to replace anyway. However, I always go back to the idea that individual teeth that are not connected are healthier and more desirable. It is easier to floss and take care of teeth that are not connected by a bridge. Implants are the number one choice in my book! If the person is a candidate for an implant, I lean in that direction, hands down.

WHAT IF YOU HAVE WORN DOWN TEETH?

If your teeth are worn down, first you need to determine why the teeth are worn down. Yes, we can fix it, but why is it happening? Let's say a person is grinding his or her teeth. You do not want to fix the teeth without knowing why the person is grinding his or her teeth because if you fix the teeth without addressing the grinding issue, the person will simply grind the fixed teeth once the procedure is completed. We may need to put the patient in a mouth guard or splint of some sort to stop the grinding. We want to make sure his or her muscles are in a relaxed state to stop the grinding cycle from happening. Most people grind in their sleep and they do not even realize it. Once you get them in a comfortable position where they are not crunching hard or grinding, then you can talk about replacing what they have lost due to this habit.

If the patient has lost a great deal of enamel and dentin tooth structure, you want to replace that with something very strong, like porcelain. If there is just a little bit of wear and tear, sometimes you can opt for bonding and reshaping the teeth. It all depends upon the level of damage. Something real extreme may require technology that is more advanced and requires more time and work to fix the damage. Most of the time, you can catch the early stage of grinding just by looking at the structure of a patient's enamel so you can diagnose the problem before it causes extreme damage.

Unfortunately, sometimes people come into my office after years of wear and tear, wondering what they can do. When this is the case, it requires something more extensive to bring someone back to full form and function. If we can catch it early, we can do something simple like a mouth guard, reshaping a few things or maybe doing a little bit of bonding. However, the first step is to figure out why this is happening and then you can talk about how you can fix it. Because we have so many options available to us today in the field of cosmetic dentistry, there is no patient that we cannot help restore her smile, give her confidence and make her happier with her appearance.

I would like to end the chapter by telling the readers about a very special young woman that I am helping right now to give her a brand new smile. The "Smile Story" is a national contest promoted by the American Academy of Cosmetic Dentistry. Contestants had to submit an application telling the AACD why they believed they should win a smile makeover. The winner of the contest was based on a social media vote. I received a call about a month ago from one of the seven contestants. She was a girl from Illinois named Amanda Kessler. Her story is quite profound. It is very emotional and it made me want to help her. I needed to submit x-rays, models and photography for the judges to consider. She came into my office and we did all this for her. She told me her story and it really tugged at my heart. I said, "Good luck. I hope that you are one of those people who will win the makeover contest." I was thrilled when I heard that she was one of the winners.

The AACD has asked me to move forward and do a complete makeover for Amanda. The AACD sent me a video camera so that I can record the process to show at our scientific conference next May in San Francisco. We are busy with Amanda right now, performing all of the work for the makeover. It is a wonderful story, with an amazing person, that people can read about on the AACD website at smilestory.com.

(This content should be used for informational purposes only. It does not create a doctor-patient relationship with any reader and should not be construed as medical advice. If you need medical advice, please contact a doctor in your community who can assess the specifics of your situation.)

6

WHO CAN BENEFIT FROM COSMETIC DENTISTRY?

by Lance Timmerman, D.M.D.

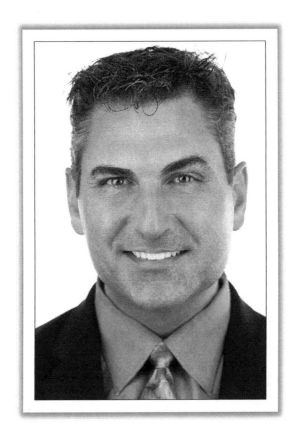

Lance Timmerman, D.M.D.

Lance Timmerman, D.M.D.
Tukwila, Washington
www.drtimmerman.com

Since 1998, cosmetic dentist Dr. Lance Timmerman DMD has been helping people in Seattle with personal, caring and advanced procedures designed to improve the health and appearance of their smiles. He has based his practice on providing his patients with personalized care. He believes in investing the time that it takes to ensure that each patient fully understands his or her condition and the treatment options. He explains everything in plain language and answers patient questions so patients can make an informed decision about the treatment plan that is right for them.

This personalized care has made Dr. Timmerman one of the top cosmetic dentists. As a facial esthetics expert, he is a leading dental provider for Botox and other injectibles and teaches other dentists. ABC affiliate KOMO 4 News did a special feature on Dr. Timmerman and his practice.

Dr. Timmerman graduated from the Oregon Health Sciences University School of Dental Medicine. He has not only learned the lessons that only experience can teach, he has continued his dental education with courses at the prestigious Las Vegas Institute for Advanced Dental Studies (LVI), NYU's Aesthetic Advantage and John Kois Center for Dental Excellence. His membership and certifications in advanced dental organizations allow him to keep current in the various aspects of dental care that matter to his patients and demonstrate his knowledge and skill.

WHO CAN BENEFIT FROM COSMETIC DENTISTRY?

The answer to that question is probably everybody. But not everybody takes advantage of the opportunity to get a smile makeover. When I first was training in this field, I assumed I was going to be seeing middle-aged to older women looking for cosmetic work. But, in terms of pure cosmetic, elective, appearance improvements, those requests come from both guys and girls, young and old. I discovered that everybody has a different motivator.

For example, a young car salesman came to us once in search of help. He was mindful of the fact that his ability to succeed was hindered by his appearance—specifically his lackluster smile. Whether we like it or not, people judge us. That first impression comes into play from the minute they meet you. Sadly, having an ugly smile says something about you that people interpret as negative. We don't know whether that first impression and the conclusions people draw from it are true or not, we just know that people draw the conclusions. The first impression an ugly smile creates is that you're either unwilling or unable to maintain your smile. And having really crooked teeth might tell them your level of intelligence is below average. There is not the first bit of evidence to support such conclusions, but some people can be very judgmental. A good healthy smile goes a long way toward creating that positive first impression.

CAN A NEW SMILE CHANGE YOUR LIFE?

A smile makeover can change your life. The same young man we were just talking about had a powerful, life-changing result. Let's call this guy Brad. As I said, Brad was a car salesman at the beginning of what he hoped would be a stellar career. Brad had played baseball as a boy and, while positioned at shortstop, took a grounder right in the teeth. They patched him up temporarily, but he didn't have any further work done on the damaged teeth. As time passed, the teeth began to decay and a root canal was necessary.

When Brad is out and about with his buddies his smile is no big deal, but when he's trying to sell high-end, luxury cars and because of his teeth, he doesn't appear to be top-of-the-line, it might create some difficulty in closing the deal. (Have you ever seen a realtor driving a beat up, fifteen-year-old Mercury? Point made.)

Brad came to me hoping to upgrade his appearance and see if that would help his career. He'd already taken all the sales training and motivational courses about how to sell cars, but it just didn't seem to be working the way he had envisioned. So we did a complete smile makeover for Brad: a combination of a few implants, some veneers, and in the end, we had transformed his smile, and unbeknownst to us, his career.

When Brad came back a few months later to have his teeth cleaned, he was able to share with us how things had gone since his smile makeover. He had actually set a new sales record at the dealership. He was convinced that his new smile gave him a deeper sense of confidence. Brad felt that the primary factor in his success was the way he felt about himself after he got his new smile. We know that Brad's skill and ability were responsible for his success, but before the new smile, he didn't often have the chance to exhibit his skills. We certainly contributed some small part to the improved career, and we are so very proud of that.

In a different case, a woman came to me who simply seemed burdened by life. She reminded me of Eeyore, the sad donkey from Winnie the Pooh. This lady, who was probably in her mid-forties, had recently gone through a divorce. She was overweight and she just wasn't a very happy person. Even though she had previously had braces and straightening done to her teeth, there were gaps growing between the teeth now that the braces were gone. The gaps were catching food between them and in addition she had big, ugly mercury fillings in her teeth and the fillings appeared gray or black.

Overall, she was the very picture of emotional and dental distress. She thought perhaps we could help.

After our assessment, she decided to have a full mouth reconstruction done. This full reconstruction was more than just a smile makeover; it involved the upper and lower teeth including her posteriors, which meant that her bite was affected also. Happily, we were able to address all her dental needs. We corrected her bite and did some reconstruction work on her teeth to close the gapping between them.

What was most interesting, though, was that when she came back months after we finished her work, she seemed genuinely happier. There she was, just beaming! She had a new boyfriend and she had lost a lot of weight, and I think probably the best word to describe her now is perky. She is just a happier person. Because of the way she felt about herself and her new confidence which somehow came with her new smile, she took control of her life, lost weight, and found a person who eventually became her new husband. That was about twelve years ago and she still gives us the majority of the credit. She believes the turning point in her life came when, because of the smile makeover, she gained the confidence to take control of her life, and that changed everything.

Everybody is different so, of course, we can never promise that cosmetic dentistry is going to increase your sales or is going to improve the selection in your dating pool. But we do make big differences in people's lives. It's very common to see patients who have trained themselves to hide their smiles because they are self-conscious. If they laugh, they bring a hand up to hide the way they look. Some never show teeth when they smile.

Some of our patients need a little crash course in smiling when we're done, because they honestly don't know how to smile.

Most of my patients come back with stories similar to these, and it makes me so proud to have the chance to make somebody else's life a little more magical.

A COSMETIC DENTIST—WHAT DOES THAT MEAN?

In the world of cosmetic dentistry, there seems to be a bit of confusion about how we define ourselves and what we do. As a matter of fact, I wouldn't be surprised if every office in the country defines its mission differently. It's no wonder, then, that some consumers are confused about the term, as well. Here's how I think of what we do: I think cosmetic dentistry is about aesthetics. We attempt to make dentistry beautiful. Old-fashioned dentistry didn't have many choices. They had to use fillings that were made from mercury amalgam that eventually turned black, leaving ugly dark spots in the patient's smile. The old model for dentistry was very functional, but it wasn't all that pretty. Someone who practices cosmetic dentistry will do a plastic composite tooth restoration, which is infinitely prettier than a metal filling. By my definition, a gold crown is okay, but when we put porcelain over it, it becomes more aesthetically pleasing.

Specifically, what we do is "smile makeovers." The patient elects to do something that will dramatically enhance his smile or her appearance — a smile makeover — something that deserves before and after photos similar to what you might find in a magazine. We create smile makeovers that transform people. Our patients want to become more glamorous and we help them do that.

When you drive down the street, you see that most dentists these days claim to do "Family and Cosmetic Dentistry." What that means is, this dentist does fillings and things that look pretty — like whitening — but he is probably neither specially trained nor sufficiently experienced to do total "smile makeovers" which are the heart and soul of Cosmetic Dentistry.

FINDING THE RIGHT COSMETIC DENTIST

Choosing a cosmetic dentist can be very confusing since most dentists will say in their marketing materials and their signage that they do "family and cosmetic dentistry." This language is a little misleading because it makes people think that they can just go anywhere and get a smile makeover. There is a lot more to cosmetic dentistry than what they teach in dental school. So, as a consumer, you must first do your homework to discover whether or not the dentist you have chosen has the training and techniques to satisfy your goals. (It's terribly important that you have clearly identified your goals. This is a big decision and it can be an expensive and long-lasting one. You want to be certain of what you want, not necessarily what you'll settle for.)

Many cosmetic dentists advertise, but word-of-mouth is the very best advertising available anywhere and it cannot be purchased. (But, do be wary of "reviews" you find online. Those CAN BE and ARE often bought and paid for.) If a patient sees a friend who had some cosmetic dentistry done and done very well, that friend is probably the best resource that patient can find for help in selecting a dentist.

To find the best cosmetic dentist with whom you feel confident, you should interview several dentists. Make an appointment to go in for a consultation. Many cosmetic dentists offer free consultations. The free consultation isn't much more than a quick discussion about what you want. We call these kinds of interviews "cocktail party consults." If you ran into me at a cocktail party and asked me questions, I could answer those questions but that certainly is nothing like an examination. I didn't look into your mouth, I didn't take x-rays, and I don't have study models. I haven't designed your case because, without all of that information I can't tell you how much it's going to cost. Of course, we cannot quote a fee until we've done the proper diagnostics, and the only way we do proper diagnostics is to do an examination. An examination and a consultation are two different things.

During your quest, you should look carefully at the dentist's education, background, and training. As you're investigating the doctor's education, don't assume that a dental license is enough. That degree simply ensures that he knows the minimum to pass the necessary exams. You need to make sure that the dentist has actually taken advanced cosmetic dental training beyond dental school.

At the risk of putting too fine a point upon it, it is critical that consumers understand this about cosmetic dentistry: Just graduating from dental school does not mean that that dentist is capable of doing cosmetic dentistry. As a matter of fact, cosmetic dentistry training isn't even something we learn in dental school. The training that makes us cosmetic dentistry experts comes from continuing education and other, more specialized programs. In order to know if your dentist has the proper training, you need to ask him where he trained specifically for cosmetics.

There are some superior training programs and, of course, some institutes are better than others. I have studied at multiple institutes in order to achieve my diverse training. You can also tell a lot about where a dentist's interests lie by looking at how he is credentialed in terms of continuing education. In medicine and in dentistry—cosmetic or otherwise—exciting changes happen every year. So, if your dentist is routinely getting more than the minimum required hours of continuing education, that's usually a sign that he is dedicated to staying up to date. But just putting in hours isn't enough. You also need to know where and when he did his cosmetic training. I, for example, have done the entire curriculum at the Las Vegas Institute for Advanced Dental Studies. Initially, I enrolled in order to learn to do porcelain veneer smile makeovers. That started me down the path to more training. I wanted to make sure that I was able to address the patient's occlusion, or the bite, as part of the entire smile makeover. That training helps the veneers last longer and, as it worked out, that led me on to other courses and eventually, through an entire curriculum.

Beyond education and extended course work, experience is also critical. Because this dentist attended classes and sat through a lecture or two on how to do a smile makeover, doesn't mean that he can do one. Experience is the second part of the lynchpin. You don't want to be a guinea pig. If your dentist just finished the cosmetic dentistry program last week, you can bet he's not as proficient as someone who completed the curriculum at LVI 15 years ago and has done hundreds of cases since. The only real way to know if he has the experience is to ask for photographs of his past cases.

Here is another important caveat: There are books produced just for dentists that are jam-packed with before-and-after photos of veneer cases. It is possible that a dentist could present just such a book on veneer cases for you to look through, without actually "saying" it's his own work. In reality, it was a book that was purchased at the last Dental Convention and not his work at all. Always ask for photo album and then ask outright if these photos are actually his own work or if it's something that was borrowed or purchased. (Don't be bashful about this. You wouldn't hire a photographer for your daughter's wedding if he had no portfolio to show you containing examples of his previous work.)

In my office, I like to go above and beyond all of that. I like to show the process to my patients. I want them to understand what's going to happen, because I want them to make a thoroughly educated decision and give us a well-founded, well-informed consent to treat. I also think it shows without a doubt that ours is not a "prep and pray method." We are definitely not like some dentists who just prep the teeth and pray that the lab gives them something pretty. I believe that the more I show the patients about the process a well-trained cosmetic dentist uses, the more at ease they'll feel going into the procedure. Additionally, it helps my patients feel as though they are in control every step of the way, and are confident that the outcome will meet their goals.

We actually have a catalog of smile styles or designs of the teeth to let the patient select the style as opposed to just me saying we'll just make the teeth longer or we'll round the corners or whatever I think is pretty. We actually show our patients on a computer screen what we plan to do; we identify the ideal proportions of the teeth which are called golden proportions. They fall into line proportionally—perfection follows rules just as Leonardo Da Vinci and the other Renaissance geniuses discovered in nature centuries ago—the Fibonacci numbers work every time. I use these tools in the process because I think it can help the patients feel confident that they've chosen a well-trained and capable dentist. The ultimate definition of success in the case of cosmetic dentistry is that the patient is happy with the end result. What is clinically perfect, or what I might think is pretty, means absolutely nothing unless the patient is happy.

COMMON COSMETIC DENTAL PROCEDURES

The Porcelain Veneer: A smile makeover will often include what we call porcelain veneers, which are also called porcelain laminate. A porcelain veneer is a layer of porcelain that covers the front surface or the part of the tooth that shows when you smile. The veneer can sometimes wrap around the sides of the teeth, or extend down the tip of the tooth or may even cover three quarters of the tooth leaving the back side or the posterior part of the tooth untouched. A full crown, on the other hand, covers the tooth completely. Put simply, a veneer is the front half of a porcelain crown.

Veneers require some preparation of the existing tooth, but not all veneers require us to do major reduction or removal of tooth structure itself. If the teeth are perfectly straight to begin with, we can be very, very conservative with the prepping of the tooth structure. Occasionally, we can avoid any prep at all. The majority of the patients we see, though, have some issue with the alignment of the tooth or something that's broken down on the tooth structure that requires some minor alteration of the surface of the tooth. This gives our lab technicians room to fabricate the porcelain veneer so that it is thick enough that it doesn't break. This also enables the technicians to blend colors to make a whiter appearance. Some people want age appropriate colors, so we don't necessarily always go bright white. This is also true if we're only doing a few of the teeth that show; we need to blend the color of the veneer so that it looks natural with adjacent teeth. Thus, having adequate latitude for the lab technician to blend colors and make it look natural often requires some removal of tooth structure. One of the advantages of the porcelain veneer is that it gives us (the lab technician and the dentist) total control of the end result.

Control of the end result is extremely important to being successful at what we do. And sometimes, in this field, more is really better. For example, if someone came in with crooked, ugly, yellow teeth; we could do braces. Afterwards, the patient would have straight, ugly, yellow teeth. We may have improved the alignment, but there might still be broken, chipped, worn and yellow teeth. Now if we just bleached the patient's crooked, ugly, yellow teeth; our patient would then have crooked, ugly, white teeth. This is the beautiful thing about porcelain veneers; we can use veneers to give the appearance of straight teeth. In the end, with veneers, we can take crooked, ugly, yellow teeth and make straight, beautiful, white teeth all at once and usually within just two visits. (The first visit is to prepare the tooth structure. The second visit is to bond the restoration into place.)

Not every patient is a candidate for veneers, but it is more possible than a lot of people think. Here's the bottom line when it comes to candidacy for veneers: if your teeth are really straight and you just want minor improvements, then we will probably recommend porcelain veneers.

If your teeth have had a lot of restoration work already, like root canals or missing tooth structures, we might suggest crowns as an answer for you. If a tooth is already missing or it had an existing bridge, we may be converting that to an implant and individual crown. In the end, though, you end up with a smile makeover. We may not be able to take a completely conservative approach because of the condition of your teeth when you came to us.

Case in point: if there is already a crown in place, it might become more difficult to add a veneer because crowns don't veneer well. In a case like that, you would be better off just replacing the old crown with a brand new one. The current condition of your teeth and your previous dental history is usually the determining factor in deciding whether or not porcelain veneers are an option for you.

We are often asked how veneers hold up over time. If they're done correctly and bonded properly, porcelain veneers hold up very, very well. In fact, the patient is probably better off than if the teeth were left untouched. Here's why. Think about a tile floor. Individual tiles can break fairly easily. But, when the tile is cemented and properly bonded to the floor, you can roll a piano over the tile and it won't break.

Having said that, I must add a word of caution: there are some dentists who are unfamiliar with bonding protocols. When a dentist doesn't know the precise way to bond a veneer to a tooth, problems can arise. The longevity of a veneer is not determined based upon the durability of the material of the veneer, but the fabrication and proper placement of the restoration to the existing tooth structure. If this isn't done well, you may get cavities around the edges. If the installation is not done well, the bonding may fail during a meal and the veneer will pop right off. None of my patients have had veneers pop off, but I've seen patients with this problem whose veneers were done elsewhere.

When a veneer pops off, the second go around is different from when the veneer was first placed. We have to limit our expectations on the second try, because when you have a fresh, brand new porcelain veneer and a freshly prepared tooth, the bonding surface is more durable. But, ultimately veneers wear well. I have replaced veneers for people who had them done 25 years before. The only reason that they are re-doing them is because, 25 years ago, the options did not include the super bright white that we offer today. So if left alone, those cases probably would have lasted maybe another decade or two. If the goal in the first place was to have a "smile makeover," the veneers of 25 years ago were a complete and continuing success. But, if your goal has changed to include a bright white smile, a second "makeover" is absolutely in order. The veneer didn't fail, the technology of a quarter-century ago did.

I had a patient who was a kick boxer. For somebody like him, all bets are off. If he gets kicked in the face and breaks a tooth, it's not the fault of the dentist or the product. In this man's case, we did the veneers for him anyway. It was nearly 11 years later when he came in with a slight crack in one of them. I wanted to remove the old veneer and bond in a new one, but it was extremely difficult to remove it. The veneer was still very smooth. If you looked hard, you could see a crack in it but the veneer wasn't really broken. Nevertheless, we wanted it to be perfect—it wasn't enough that you would have to strain your eyes in order to tell that there was a crack there. My point is, these veneers are very, very strong, but they are not bullet-proof.

Missing Teeth: We tell our patients that there are really only four choices if they have missing teeth.

1. *Do Nothing:* It is perfectly acceptable to do nothing. However, you should understand that there are consequences for doing nothing. There are some consequences that come into play immediately like aesthetic issues, and some that come over time, such as what happens when your other teeth begin to migrate and move out of place. This is not just a problem of there being more space between your teeth, but in time, medical issues can develop if you're not able to chew your food properly.

2. *Partial Denture:* The next step up would be what we call a partial denture or even a full denture depending how many teeth are missing. If you're missing just one or two teeth, a partial denture may work just fine for you. A partial denture is an appliance that's usually removable and has a false tooth attached to it. It's something that fills the gap in your smile and acts to hold the other teeth in place. Nevertheless, I need to say that 99 percent of my patients who have partial dentures actually hate them. They almost always want to do something different when the time is right. (This means when they need something different physically or can better afford the change.)

3. *A Bridge:* A step up from a partial denture is a bridge. A bridge can be a fixed or non-removable appliance. We use the teeth adjacent to the missing tooth to support or to anchor a restoration piece that includes a replacement for the missing tooth as part of the whole.

It works like this: If you had one missing tooth, we reduce the tooth structure on either side of that missing tooth, as we would if we were going to do a full crown. Then, instead of having an individual crown, we would fuse the three teeth together with a single new restoration that included all three. A triple crown, if you will. Generally, this works very well but the problem with this particular solution is durability. For example, if you get a cavity on one of the teeth that anchors your bridge, the entire bridge would have to be replaced. Unfortunately, the reason you may develop a cavity in that particular spot is that it's more challenging to floss under the bridge. Some people have trouble managing even to brush their teeth adequately, let alone floss in a difficult-to-reach area. That neglect can lead to bone loss around the supporting teeth or cavities around the supporting teeth and in the end, this means the entire bridge has to be replaced.

4. ***Dental Implants:*** The best option we turn to when we're dealing with missing teeth is dental implants. Dental implants open up additional options for people who would otherwise be destined for dentures of some kind, whether partial dentures or full dentures. We do lots of implants in our office. They can actually help us save virgin teeth—teeth that have never been touched— never had a cavity and are in really good shape. Virgin teeth would have to be prepped in order to be used to support a bridge. Instead of ruining those virgin teeth, we implant a man-made root into the jaw bone where the tooth is missing, then attach a restoration on top of the implant. This attachment can be done with cement or by screwing the restoration into place. With this method, we

can place a single crown, or in cases where an entire arch of teeth is missing, we can place several implants in order to support a fixed bridge. These implanted restorations, then, are more or less permanent, meaning you won't be treating them like a removable appliance. They are there to stay. You treat them just as you do your own teeth.

As far as durability for these four options, the longevity runs in essentially the same order. A partial denture is not as durable because it depends upon the adjacent teeth to support it. There are attachments or hooks that attach to adjacent teeth but because the appliance is coming in and out of the mouth all the time, it creates a different set of problems. This appliance is put on and taken off daily. This movement affects the existing teeth by creating torsion or torque on the adjacent teeth. Constant pushing and pulling upon the healthy teeth can eventually make them weak and they can come out. Once those healthy teeth come out, the partial is no longer any good. Now you need to make another partial using a different tooth for support. That new one will torque, then that one will come out, and then you need another new partial; and so the story goes on.

With a bridge, you still have tooth structure in place. As we mentioned before, you might be forced to replace the bridge because of tooth decay. In some cases, during the process of creating the bridge, your nerve becomes injured. If the nerve dies, you'll need a root canal and when that happens you need to have a new partial.

Implants, on the other hand, have some major advantages. You cannot get a cavity on an implant. You can't get periodontal disease without a periodontal ligament, and implants don't have periodontal ligaments. With well-placed and well-cared-for implants, you can actually preserve bone that exists and prevent further bone loss. Dental implants are really the longest-lasting restoration we have in dentistry today.

Whitening: When we talk about smile makeovers, we have to discuss tooth color. Interestingly, for many people who come to us initially considering cosmetic dentistry, the most important part of the entire process is the color of their smile. They seem oblivious to the fact that the alignment of their teeth is not attractive, or that their teeth are worn down. Their first concern is the color. I suspect this is because there are entire industries sprouting up around the concept of tooth color. You can't pick up a magazine or turn on the television without hearing about whiter teeth.

In my estimation, there are only three main factors people need to consider when it comes to whitening teeth:

1. There will always be some sort of gel or peroxide formulation.

2. The concentration of the gel formulation and the frequency with which you will be doing the applications. Will it be a one-time-only application or once daily for several weeks?

3. Duration. Will you be using the gel for an hour or for 8 hours?

Each one of these factors is going to have a significant impact upon the final results.

All tooth whitening programs are not created equal. It's unreasonable to expect somebody who treated her teeth one time for 15 minutes, to have the same results as someone who treated her tooth structure with highly concentrated gel eight hours a day for three weeks.

As I mentioned, the concentration of hydrogen peroxide is a critical factor in whitening one's teeth. The legal limit for hydrogen peroxide tooth whitener is nine percent over the counter at the drugstore. In the dentist's office, we can go to a higher concentration. Some very common concentrations of take-home gel for whitening purposes are anywhere from 15 to 22 percent. If the treatment is an in-office procedure, the concentration is usually going to be more in the 22- to 45-percent range. The whitening products we use in the office have a much higher concentration of hydrogen peroxide, so the use must be supervised by a dentist.

The higher concentrations can lead to irritation of the supporting gum tissues, and so we will often paint a barrier on to the gum tissues in order to prevent collateral damage. There are also in-office whitening procedures that use some sort of light to heat up and activate the gel more intensely. Interestingly, there is debate in dental circles about whether the light is necessary or not. There are products in the marketplace that have a high concentration and must be supervised by the dentist in a dental office, but they don't use the light and they work very well.

I think it goes without saying that if you want your teeth to be the very whitest they can possibly be, you're probably not going to get that result in a take-home bag like a free party favor from the dentist down the block. It will require having a dentist supervise the process. In our office, we incorporate a combination of in-office and at-home use. The combining of the two allows us to get the teeth intensely white and that effect lasts a very long time. The deeper we can get the whitening ingredients to penetrate into the tooth structure itself, the longer that result will last. But—in the interest of truth in advertising— all whitening is considered temporary. The whitening process will reverse itself if you don't maintain it.

As I said before, though, it's the combination of the three things—the gel concentration, the frequency, and duration of the process—that will give you the result you are looking for. Before a person starts the whitening process, we need to identify her goals in advance. Does she just want brighter teeth? If that's the case then just about any product will work. But if she wants her teeth to be transformed into the whitest white possible, then it will take a higher concentration of whitening product, applied in the dental office.

There are some things to watch out for and to understand before you start the whitening process. First of all, a tooth might have already had a dental restoration. If it's had a filling, for example, the filling won't change color. So if the filling shows when you smile or when you're looking at the tooth, and if that filling blends in really, really well with the tooth structure, then the filling may be fairly obvious if you have a dramatic shift in color. So, if you want that restored tooth to match, it may require that the filling in question be replaced after the whitening process is over. One of the best things about porcelain as a dentistry material is that it has incredible color stability. This means that if the tooth has a porcelain crown from previous dental work, it's not going to change color through the whitening process. If you have a dramatic whitening of the surrounding teeth, you may need to consider getting a new, matching crown. If you had a single front tooth restored to match your other teeth perfectly and you decide to bleach your teeth later, then that front tooth will no longer match. At that point, you will probably want to replace that crown.

People who are planning to do a combination of whitening and tooth restoration have a specific goal in mind as to how white they want the result to be. They opt to do the dental restoration first then whiten to match. The problem with this is that we can never predict how well the teeth will change color because everybody is unique. There is simply no reliable way to predict exactly how the teeth will respond. In our practice, we always suggest doing the whitening first and then making the restoration match the tooth color after the whitening process is completed. If however, the end result of that whitening is not satisfactory after we've maxed out the whitening options, then it may mean that, in order to attain your smile makeover goal, you may have to go to a different restorative option—porcelain veneers, crowns, or some combination of the two.

Another consideration is this: if there is decay present, the sensitivity in and around that decayed tooth can be increased during the whitening process. We try to address the decay first and then whiten, in order to stop the sensitivity issue before it starts. One needs to be aware, as we mentioned earlier, those restorations we do to proactively deal with sensitivity may need to be redone because of the new color.

In terms of the whitening process, there will always be some level of sensitivity. It happens because peroxides in the whitening medium penetrate deeply into the tooth structure and it results in some dehydration of the tooth. The early sensitivity that patients feel is one hundred percent reversible if it's related to that dehydration. One caveat: If the tooth is already pathologic, meaning that the nerve is already in the process of dying, the whitening process may deal that nerve a final blow and it dies. That cannot be reversed. That tooth will require restorative or dental care including, perhaps, a root canal.

That said, if the teeth are otherwise fine and healthy and there is no other pathology present, some sensitivity following the whitening process is nothing to worry about. The patient and his or her teeth are going to be fine. The process will reverse itself, and the sensitivity will go away as the tooth rehydrates. In the end, the patient has a spectacularly white smile with no sensitivity associated with the process.

There are products on the market today we can use to help prevent the sensitivity or minimize and mitigate the sensitivity a patient feels. Of course our goal is always to make the whitening process a more comfortable one. But it is probably unrealistic for the patient to expect or for the dentist to promise no sensitivity whatsoever.

We do everything we can to minimize any discomfort for our patients, but despite our efforts, there are simply some people who will experience some sensitivity and will require a little extra effort. That extra effort can mean that the process will just take a little longer. If we're planning on the patient wearing trays for two weeks but after one day he (or she) is uncomfortable enough that he cannot do the same treatment the next day, we say, "Okay, use the trays every other day." The process might take longer, but we will still be able to get the teeth whiter.

THE BITE—PRACTICAL CONCERN

When a patient is thinking about a smile makeover and is concentrating on the aesthetics of a new, stunning smile, he doesn't often take his bite into account. As dentists, we must factor this into account, no matter what else we're doing. Having the most amazing smile isn't worth much if you cannot use your teeth as they were meant to be used. They aren't just jewels—they are also tools. Their functionality is critical to your health, so we need to correctly address your bite no matter if we're doing a restoration, dental implants, or some combination of other work to create your smile makeover.

If all we're doing is veneers on the two front teeth, it really doesn't require the dentist to understand much about the bite or the mechanics of the occlusion. But as soon as we start doing several teeth at once, being able to manage the bite, the occlusion, becomes very, very important. A case involving two teeth isn't as difficult as 8 to 10 teeth and that is not nearly as difficult as all 28 teeth. The more complex your smile makeover is going to be, the more careful you must be to find a dentist who can deliver the cosmetic result as well as the functionality you absolutely need.

(This content should be used for informational purposes only. It does not create a doctor-patient relationship with any reader and should not be construed as medical advice. If you need medical advice, please contact a doctor in your community who can assess the specifics of your situation.)

7

FINDING THE RIGHT COSMETIC DENTIST REQUIRES SOME RESEARCH

by Todd C. Snyder, D.D.S.

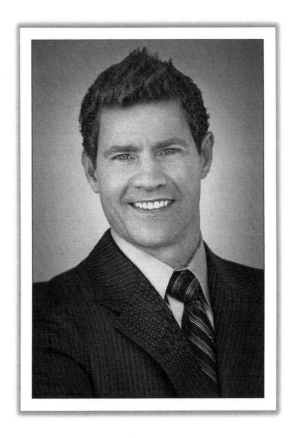

Todd C. Snyder, D.D.S.
Aesthetic Dental Designs
Orange County, California
www.aestheticdentaldesigns.com

Dr. Todd C. Snyder received his doctorate in dental surgery at the University of California at Los Angeles School of Dentistry. Thereafter, he trained at the prestigious F.A.C.E. Institute for complex gnathological and temporomandibular joint disorders (TMD). He was on the faculty of the Center for Esthetic Dentistry at U.C.L.A. where he helped create and co-direct the first every two year graduate program in Aesthetic and Cosmetic Restorative Dentistry. Dr. Snyder is currently on the faculty at Esthetic Professionals. Due to his vast experience and expertise in cosmetic dentistry, Dr. Snyder is a consultant for dental manufacturing companies and has researched and recommended changes for many of the materials now being used in dentistry.

As a dentist, author, international lecturer, researcher and instructor at various teaching facilities, Dr. Snyder offers a lot on many levels to not only his patients but also his colleagues around the world. He has authored numerous articles worldwide on contemporary restorative and cosmetic dentistry. Dr. Snyder is a member of the Catapult Elite Group, an international speaker's consortium.

Dr. Snyder is an Accredited Member of the prestigious American Academy of Cosmetic Dentistry, less than 1% of US dentists have achieved this status. His commitment to his patients goes above and beyond simply being a dentist. His comprehensive approach to cosmetic dentistry shows in the beautiful smiles that he creates.

FINDING THE RIGHT COSMETIC DENTIST REQUIRES SOME RESEARCH

When searching for a dentist who can truly transform your smile and change how you feel about yourself inside and out, you'll likely steer toward the term "cosmetic dentist" in your hunt through Google. Unfortunately, the results will reveal pretty much any dentist who has "cosmetic" listed anywhere on his or her site and won't cull them down to actual qualified, certified experts in cosmetic dentistry. Since cosmetic dentistry is not a specialty, any dentist can claim to be a cosmetic dentist even though he or she has had no additional training or expertise in the field. Accredited cosmetic dentists have completed substantial amounts of training, alongside peer reviews, to ensure that they perform high-quality cosmetic treatments.

Certainly general dentists can perform certain types of cosmetic procedures, and there are plenty of competent practitioners who can help you have a healthy, beautiful smile. But those who seek quality, lasting results for smiles that require more than a simple whitening need to carefully investigate the training and experience of dentists who claim to be "cosmetic specialists."

I have taught at the University of California, Los Angeles (UCLA) for five years, doing hands-on training with existing dentists as well as dental students. I created a two-year post-graduate education program in cosmetic dentistry that is the first of its kind in the world. I lecture internationally, as well as write articles in dental publications around the world, explaining various techniques and procedures to other dental practitioners.

When searching for a cosmetic dentist, try to find a dentist who has been accredited by a reputable dental academy or association, such as the American Academy of Cosmetic Dentistry (AACD). Before you can be accredited by the AACD, you must pass numerous tests: written, verbal, and peer-reviewed cosmetic cases. Currently, there are fewer than 400 AACD accredited dentists. Finding someone with this extra level of expertise should be a top priority in your search.

The AACD website allows you to search for one of their accredited dentists who practices near your home. There are four levels of membership in the AACD. A Fellow is the highest level of accreditation, followed by regular accredited members, and then dentists who are pursuing accreditation. On the last tier are individuals who are simply members of the organization and are not pursuing any type of accreditation. The AACD site will allow you to search by accreditation level, which should be an important consideration for you in your search.

If there are no AACD dentists in your area, check with other organizations that offer similar accreditations to cosmetic dentists. If a dentist has invested the time to go through the numerous steps to become accredited with one of these organizations, it speaks highly of the dentist's caliber. Personal references from trusted people are invaluable, so talk to any family or friends who have recently improved their smiles. Also, previous patients are good sources because they can impart a lot of the information that you may want to know but may not feel comfortable asking the dentist. Patients can give you an idea of the level of care they received such as personal information about the process, their happiness after the fact, and how the procedure has changed their lives.

Once you identify a few prospective cosmetic dentists, research their backgrounds and schedule a consultation with each one so you can compare each dentist's recommendations and procedures against your goals. A beautiful office and a nice personality are great to have, and many dentists can perform simple veneers and crowns. However, there is much more to cosmetic dentistry. It's important to understand a dentist's level of training and experience along with the number of cases they've handled that are similar to yours and whether or not they've trained other practitioners. I think that the more a person meets with various dentists, the more he or she understands the variety of approaches to cosmetic dentistry.

Don't rush the process—your smile is an important part of who you are and how you feel every day. Take the time to meet with several different dentists to find one with a high degree of skill: one who will be meticulous with each step of the process and not rush you through it. Many of my patients over the years have told me they appreciate the level of detail I employ to ensure a perfect final outcome.

ADDRESSING THE ARCHITECTURE OF YOUR FACE AND TEETH

I equate the process to building a home. After you sit down and look at different examples of exteriors and pick the style of house you want, an architect (the dentist) then develops a blueprint incorporating these concepts using his training and expertise so you can see how the final product will look. In the initial cosmetic process, you will look at different types of teeth and smiles to visualize the level of aesthetics you want for your mouth. A good dentist will then make a mock-up of that image so you can see if this is truly what you want.

Realistic teeth have a lot of character compared to very white, "Hollywood" teeth. Some people will want a realistic smile, while others want the super white, very straight, movie-star smile. In order to get the end result that the patient wants, everyone must be on the same page. The patient, dentist, and ceramist must all be on board to create the appearance the patient desires. Taking the time to set up a blueprint and visualize the final product before beginning the dental work will produce the greatest results. It's important to find a dentist who involves you in decisions and keeps you informed and educated throughout the process.

146

Cosmetic dentistry utilizes different materials, technology, techniques, and insights when evaluating a patient's teeth, smile, and gums. Teeth are not the only element involved in smile transformations. This process begins with evaluating the whole face and assessing how a new smile will fit into it. This takes extra time and effort to ensure that we get it right. Good dentists want see how a potential new look will fit your face before beginning to make changes to your teeth.

Knowing what brought the patient to the point of seeking cosmetic dentistry is very important, whether their mirror reflects gaps, chips, worn teeth, or discolored restorations, etc. I view it like a cosmetic investigation: at the end of the process, I should know how the patient got to this point and why he or she is in my office. In many cases, there is a functional aspect in addition to an appearance problem with the teeth. It can be developmental. More often than not, some type of functional problem has given the teeth their current appearance. Figuring out what caused the teeth to appear the way they do is important because the imbalance will continue to cause problems if it is not addressed. We must look at the function as well as all of the other elements before beginning to alter the teeth.

Addressing the architecture of the face and teeth is a very important step that should give the patient a long-lasting and sustainable result. Dental procedures performed without careful consideration of all contributing factors can begin to fail and turn into a new problem because the original reason why the teeth were damaged or not aesthetically pleasing was never addressed. We can change the appearance of the teeth very easily. To get the teeth to a maintainable level, we must understand the hidden causes along with the appearance of the teeth.

As a dentist, you can actually give a patient the equivalent of a facelift or plastic surgery because teeth influence the adjacent facial tissues. By bringing teeth forward or moving them out laterally, we can change the appearance of a person's smile as well as the appearance of the entire face. In one case, our patient had numerous wrinkles and a shortened lower facial height, meaning that the lower jaw and nose area looked too close together. When we finished treating the teeth, the patient had less tension in her face and her wrinkles were not as pronounced. This made her appear to look happier and more youthful. It is amazing to see the transformation that cosmetic dentistry can have on the entire face.

There are many different ways to repair the tooth to allow for better position and shape and a hundred different types of porcelain veneers and ceramic crowns on the market. The name brand isn't as important as the artistry of a highly trained, skilled dentist and a master ceramist working together with a final vision in mind. That vision closes gaps and changes the contours of the teeth, creating the amazing smile makeover that the patient desires. With veneers and crowns, you can instantly improve large amounts of tooth structure by covering the front, the side, or the whole of the tooth with ceramic. Craftsmanship, skill, and artistry are necessary to make truly amazing smiles that enhance the appearance of a person's face.

Dentists use cosmetic bonding to make a tooth with some minor wear look every bit as good (or better) as a natural tooth. This is based on the technique, the dentist, and the materials. Bonding can be used to cover the entire front of the tooth, the entire tooth, and in between teeth. The only downside of bonding is the extra time involved with the patient because all of the necessary artistry and skill used by the dentist. The teeth are the canvas a dentist works on when he uses bonding materials to correct problems. The end result is often beautiful, especially if the dentist is skilled, but it takes a substantial amount of time to do things properly.

With ceramics, the master ceramist uses all of his artistry and skill in the laboratory while the patient wears a temporary restoration. This is in alternative to the patient sitting in the chair while a dentist takes the time to create fabrications from bonding material. There are two advantages of using ceramics versus cosmetic bonding. Ceramics are less time-consuming than bonding materials, and the dentist's level of skill and talent does not have to be very high. Furthermore, different techniques can be overlapped or used in conjunction to create the smile that the patient desires. Some teeth can be restored with bonding materials while others can be restored with ceramics, based on the level of damage in each individual tooth. However, because it takes a higher level of skill to blend together ceramics, plastics, and/or bonding materials, not many dentists can do this successfully. An experienced, skilled dentist can combine any of these techniques to conservatively restore teeth—rather than destroying a lot of the tooth structure—to create that ideal perfect smile.

In addition to restorations, you can improve a person's smile by modifying the gum tissues and/or the structure of the teeth. For example, we can modify the "gummy" smiles of patients and give them more of a natural and aesthetic appearance. We begin by looking at the support of the face, along with the architecture of the gum and bone—your lips, gums, facial features. Bones establish the frame for your smile. Sometimes the gum and bone must be modified to provide the best possible result. I have seen numerous cases in which a dentist has simply fixed the teeth without bothering to address underlying issues involving the gums, bones, and lips. It made a huge difference in the end results because the dentist failed to address all of these issues when evaluating the patients for cosmetic procedures.

Once a dentist has the ideal lip-to-gum-to-bone proportion, he can begin to look at the patient's teeth. It does not matter if the patient has small teeth that have worn and shifted because the shape of the tooth can be changed in many ways with many different products and materials. Whether it is something as minimally invasive as whitening and contouring the teeth to make them look perfect, or something more extensive (such as bonding, veneers, ceramic crowns, modern implants, bridges), many different cosmetic tools can be used to alter the appearance of the teeth to enhance the smile.

The dentist must have a high level of skill and talent to perform less invasive restorations. It is much more challenging to create a great smile with less space in which to work. The dentist must also team up with a master ceramist who can create thin materials with a wonderful appearance. A less skilled dentist will need to take away more of the tooth structure to open up more room to work in order to achieve the same result as a more skilled dentist using less space. Once that tooth structure is removed, you can never get it back. Also, more lost tooth structure increases the potential for sensitivity and the risk for other treatments such as root canals. If a dentist minimizes the work by using mock-ups and other tools, this becomes a huge advantage for the patient as far as the health and maintenance of the teeth in the long term. Cosmetic work done incorrectly can result in the patient losing teeth due to irreversible damage or removed tooth structure, so that it will become necessary to install implants, bridges, or partial dentures. Some of these procedures can be avoided with a minimally invasive or "contact lens" approach.

PLANNING PHASES TO HELP YOU VISUALIZE THE END RESULTS

Since I want to ensure that my patients are happy with the end results, I use several tools during the planning phases to help my patient visualize what he or she will look like after we finish the cosmetic work. Digital photographs are useful in the planning stage because we can change our plan until we get the end result you desire, and it helps me to see potential limitations and problems as I try to restore the appearance of your smile. After we digitally achieve the desired look, we transfer that information to diagnostic models that are mounted on an "articulator." These models, using an articulator, replicate the patient's jaw movement, position, and shape so that we can judge the function of the restorations.

Most models in 90% or more of dental offices are placed on inexpensive, disposable, plastic-based mounts that do not replicate a person's jaw movement in any way, shape, or form. It is a fast, inexpensive way to create models and does not replicate jaw movement the way an articulator can. Potentially, this shortcut technique can introduce a lot of error into the final restorations and the overall appearance of a patient's smile.

Articulators have different levels of accuracy. On the first level are disposable, plastic articulators that operate like a hinge and do not replicate any of the patient's jaw movements. The next level includes the metal or metal–carbon-fiber articulators that replicate the average patient's movement. There are even higher degrees of accuracy based on the type of articulator that gets attached to a patient's head to capture information about his or her jaw movements. Based on the level of the device used, enough information can be generated to program an articulator and the actual movements of a specific patient can be replicated. Although this high-level type of articulator is not used by many dentists because of the extra time involved, this level of accuracy creates the best possible outcome. We can create the ideal movement of that patient that results in the best possible teeth to go in that particular mouth. However, many dentists use less accurate devices to save time and money, and the shortcuts result in more problems.

Using an accurate articulator is critical when you are changing a substantial amount of the tooth structure, but most patients do not know that there are different levels of accuracy. During the initial consultation, the patient should ask the dentist, "What type of articulators are you using for my case?" Is the dentist using a plastic disposable articulator or an articulator based on the average natural human dentition movement or a fully adjustable articulator?

Probably 50 to 60 percent of my work involves replacing older cosmetic dentistry that is failing or wearing down with time or recently performed cosmetic work that is failing because the dentist did not follow all of the important initial steps to determine a proper plan. Many dental processes get re-done because patients are unhappy with the final appearance, the function is bad, or the gum tissues are irritated due to bulky restorations that are too far below the gum line. The dentist who jumps in and begins work on the same day the patient schedules the appointment typically provides results that are less than satisfactory for the patient. A dentist who begins a case without planning—without using diagnostic models on highly accurate articulators, without doing mock-ups and/or jaw evaluation protocols over the course of a few weeks—is doing a disservice to clients.

In order to make sure that the dentist knows the goal and the patient knows what she wants, I do mock-ups and get the patient involved with the preliminary work. The patients themselves can help create the ideal smile, as this is not a one-sided process. It involves discovering what you want and see as an ideal smile as well as educating you on what is considered cosmetically pleasing and what the realistic possibilities are given your current circumstances. Another advantage of using a mock-up of the teeth is that the dentist gains more insight as to the amount of the tooth structure that needs to be reduced. It takes a higher level of skill and difficulty to create something less invasive as opposed to simply cutting away tooth structure to install ceramics.

Sometimes, dentists need to evaluate patients over a week or a few months to get the patient's teeth and jaw bones into a position that allows for better restoration longevity. In some cases, a dentist may need to correct function first to eliminate or reduce the primary causes of wear, damage, or tooth movement that has prompted the need for a smile to be rebuilt. By addressing the function it may be possible to minimize or prevent future breakage, leakage, and tooth movement due to placing the new restorations in a better, less stressful position within the mouth. If this is not addressed, then the new restoration could have earlier failure due to damage from fatigue pressure, or it may have earlier adhesive failure. If the dentist is not using highly accurate articulators or not evaluating the job properly, the patient could receive below-standard cosmetic services.

When you are comparing ceramic to bonding and deciding which technique is preferable, it actually depends more on the type of problem that needs to be resolved rather than comparing the materials to each other. If the dentition needs to be fixed for just an individual tooth, using ceramics may mean that the laboratory technician will need a couple of attempts to get it looking good. This means that a patient will have to visit the office a few times. Eventually, with a good master ceramist, you can get something that matches the adjacent teeth perfectly.

Unfortunately, many dentists and ceramists who cannot match one tooth will start to cut down adjacent healthy teeth to create a uniform appearance when using ceramics. Taking away healthy tooth structure is not an ideal solution for creating a natural look on one damaged tooth. Bonding can often be a better alternative. With the right amount of skill and artistry, dentists can create a single tooth from bonding that looks every bit as good as the adjacent teeth, without damaging any of the adjacent tooth structure. In the right circumstances, bonding can be just as durable and can hold up just as well as ceramics.

Based on the size of the defect, ceramics have slightly better durability when compared to bonding, which is really a plastic. It's better to use bonding for smaller defects because bonding is less invasive and can fix a small hole without causing a lot of damage. For larger restorations on multiple teeth, ceramics are typically better than bonding. However, bonding is not as color-stable. After eight to ten years, you might begin seeing some color changes. If ceramics are not scratched or polished with abrasive agents, ceramics can maintain their color much longer than bonding. Of course, every material has limited longevity based on the patient's hygiene, diet, and function. Eventually, everything will need to be replaced.

If a dentist avoids damaging or removing the tooth structure, he has more opportunities to make needed repairs to the teeth in the future. That is often one of the advantages in using bonding. In some patient cases, we did bonding on ten of the upper front teeth and six of the lower front teeth. After eight years, these teeth still looked amazing and had great color. However, that is not always the best approach based on the patient's function. Some people may start to break things earlier, so it's more advantageous to install a more durable product. Based on the necessary amount of time that goes into using bonding, along with considerations of color and time and durability, clients may opt to use more durable ceramics instead. Ceramics can occasionally in some cases be placed with very minimal to no adjustment of tooth structure.

THE BENEFITS OF COSMETIC DENTISTRY

A nice smile is important for many reasons, which is why doing mock-ups beforehand becomes critical. The patient and dentist can evaluate the smile before the work begins. It is amazing how a patient's face lights up and looks more youthful when she is happy with her smile. Changing your smile changes your physical appearance and even your personality. You can just tell when a person feels better about himself because he is more confident, outgoing, and happier.

Some research shows that more opportunities arise for jobs and relationships when a person has a better smile, a better outlook on life, and a better feeling about himself. Having an improved appearance or a more attractive smile opens the doors to so many other opportunities. I would say that this is very important in creating the best opportunities and enjoyment for a person's life.

When you have a job interview, you dress to impress and want to look your best; and one of the first things people notice is your smile. The same idea about displaying the best possible appearance applies when you are meeting someone at church, at the grocery store, or at a restaurant. A great smile can help in many ways. Look at all of the people in Hollywood that we admire. Why do we idolize them or see them the way that we do? Why are we constantly looking through magazines with these people on the cover? It is because of their appearance and achievements which typically includes a great smile.

You do not see many celebrities with crooked or irregular teeth. Many people first turn to plastic surgery to improve their appearance, though I could show them many examples of cases in which the teeth were changed first and that made a huge difference. Altering the teeth first can save people money, time, and the discomfort of a plastic surgery procedure. While plastic surgery can be transformational, teeth should be reviewed first to see if the desired change can be achieved without it. The importance of an attractive smile has been documented to show substantial benefits in a person's career and relationships. That alone speaks volumes as to why people should consider cosmetic dentistry.

I cannot say enough wonderful things about the show Extreme Makeover. The show increased the public's understanding about the possible and dramatic changes that cosmetic dentistry can make to change a person's appearance and life. It was wonderful to see how those patients' faces would light up after they saw the results. I get to see that every day—it is a wonderful experience to be a part of changing someone's life. The best part is when you hand a patient a mirror and she gets to see how she looks. Sometimes she is just overwhelmed with emotion and joy. I can think of two recent examples in which my office helped to change someone's life through cosmetic dentistry.

A divorced, unemployed teacher came into the office. She had very short, worn down, small teeth. Her lower facial height, from her nose to her chin, was scrunched up and tight when she smiled. Her face had a lot of tension, so she had many wrinkles. Her neck was very tight; ligaments popped up from her neck when she smiled. She tried to hide her excessively gummy and bony smile by not smiling very big or very often. Changing all of her teeth and smile showed an amazing transformation, especially since we were able to get her face to relax so she could smile bigger. She said that it took her a while to actually feel comfortable with her new smile because she had always been accustomed to hiding her teeth. It took her some time to realize that she could smile big and did not need to hide anything anymore.

The before-and-after photos of her face were just amazing. The tension was gone, her face was smooth and relaxed, and all of those weird neck wrinkles and protrusions just vanished. She looked so much younger and happier, with a wonderful presence about her. We literally caused a change in her personality in addition to changing the appearance of her face and smile. She has since remarried, had children, and is now teaching at a university. She equates all of this being happier and more confident because of her new smile.

Another patient was an engineer who could not smile. He had substantially worn teeth, and his face was also scrunched up with many wrinkles from wear and tear and muscle tension. He had gaps between his teeth, many of which were cracked, chipped, and worn down. He had an asymmetric, weird smile. With time, we were able to get his jaw into the right position. We changed the shape of all of his teeth by making them longer, and then whitened his teeth.

His metamorphosis over time was just incredible, as if he had gone through plastic surgery. He lost 10 to 15 years just in the appearance of his face. After the fact, he told us that he used to have facial muscle tension and discomfort and some ear ringing problems. All of these problems went away after the dentistry was performed. He said that he would finally be able to smile. When we asked, he said, "Yes, it was very difficult to smile back then." The muscles hurt and it was almost impossible for him to smile. After his procedures, his face looked more youthful—it was just amazing.

After his dental work was completed, our patient's company grew and expanded. As the head of the company, there were many business meetings that required him to talk to people about opportunities. He told us how much the company had grown and that he felt it was all due to him being happy and healthy, but also looking and feeling good because of the smile change. He said it was the best investment he had ever made.

FIND A DENTIST WHO WILL SIT DOWN AND DISCUSS YOUR OPTIONS

Our office is rather unique in taking a substantial amount of time to sit with our patients and talk to them about possibilities, evaluating things so that they get a better understanding of what can be done. We offer complimentary consultations to all of our patients for cosmetic procedures. I explain the different techniques that we employ to figure out what we can do to enhance the patient's smile. At the same time, I explain to my patients that I want them involved to ensure their satisfaction with the final result. If the patients don't know what they want, we can show them options to help them figure out exactly what they desire from a smile makeover.

It takes a lot of time and effort to achieve the best result. Explaining to a patient what is possible and what we can do for them speaks volumes about how we conduct our practice. I believe that is why we see people wanting to work with us from all over the world. The time that we take to investigate and get it right sets us apart. We show you options, get you involved to find out what you will like, and create it for you. Many patients benefit from our level of expertise, education, and training.

We help patients obtain a better appearance by using minimally invasive techniques, such as teeth whitening or minor contouring of the teeth, to something with a little more effect, like cosmetic bonding. Sometimes we move on to larger procedures, such as porcelain veneers, crowns, and implants. Depending on each patient's mouth, we offer different options, from minimally invasive or non-invasive protocols to more extensive procedures. There is no one out there who cannot derive some benefit from enhancing his current smile. I believe that our meticulous attention to detail, our skill and artistry, as well as the master ceramists that we use, is not often seen in dentistry today. Many dentists are more focused on insurance concerns and the need to increase patients in order to increase revenue than on the quality of work.

For me, helping people and creating opportunities for them by giving them a beautiful smile is extremely rewarding and even fun. I really enjoy spending time with them to make them feel better about themselves, to create better opportunities for them by giving them the best possible outcome. I love doing this! It is not just my job. I really get a lot of pleasure from helping my clients. Therefore, I am meticulous and take everything to a very high level of accuracy and detail. In my lectures and articles, I relate all of the little things that are often missing in modern dentistry, which is one of the many reasons why we achieve substantially better outcomes for our patients. Patients would be happier with longer-lasting, less invasive, more functional restorations. They just need to find a cosmetic dentist who takes the time to properly evaluate the patient and the patient's needs before beginning any cosmetic procedure or treatment.

(This content should be used for informational purposes only. It does not create a doctor-patient relationship with any reader and should not be construed as medical advice. If you need medical advice, please contact a doctor in your community who can assess the specifics of your situation.)

8

WHEN WE CHANGE YOUR SMILE, IT CAN CHANGE YOUR LIFE FOREVER

by Mary Swift, D.D.S.

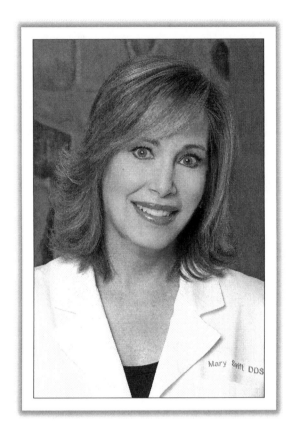

Mary Swift, D.D.S.
Dallas Laser Dentistry
Dallas, Texas
www.dallascosmeticdentistry.us

With over 30 years in the dental profession, Texas General Dentist Dr. Mary Swift is known for her advanced dental and cosmetic techniques, which she continues to improve with hundreds of post-graduate course hours. Dr. Swift and her staff have received the Consumer's Choice Award for Cosmetic Dentistry the last four years. After being trained in 2004 in the use of BOTOX® to treat TMJ headache pain, she became nationally renowned.

Dr. Mary Swift founded Dallas Laser Dentistry in 1997. Her focus on patient service has helped change the way modern private practice dentistry operates in Dallas. Her patients relax in a soothing, spa-like environment overlooking North Dallas, complete with heated massage chairs and aromatherapy, while Dr. Mary Swift utilizes her extensive experience, laser technology, advanced training and aesthetic skills to analyze and create a smile uniquely designed and ideally suited to the patient's face.

With her patients, Dr. Swift is known for her caring and educational approach, her ability to listen to each patient's desires, for involving each patient in the development of their own unique treatment plan and for her customized smile creations that optimize each patient's facial bone structure and personality. Dr. Swift builds smiles that not only are contagious, but that are designed to last.

WHEN WE CHANGE YOUR SMILE, IT CAN CHANGE YOUR LIFE FOREVER

Cosmetic dentistry can help a patient in terms of self-esteem and confidence. Our judgmental society does not take long to form an opinion about another person, whether that opinion is correct or not, and that judgment is often solely based on an appearance-based image. Recently, a 29-year-old man (we will call him Jessie) came into my office for a consultation. I love consultations—I do not charge for them. I love to listen to what patients have been told by other dentists as well as learn about the patient and his perspective. In my office, Jessie told me that he was advancing in his career but felt as if he was not being taken seriously. He wanted to know what we could do to change his smile.

Jessie's nice, healthy teeth also had spaces in between almost all of his front teeth, both top and bottom. Most of the time when people think about spaces between teeth, they think about kids. That's why Jessie felt he was not being taken seriously. Our office performed image consulting, showing him what his smile would look like once we corrected the spaces. With the spaces filled in, Jessie appeared more mature, so he followed through with the treatment and has since gotten the promotion that he wanted.

When people see someone with teeth that are stained, dark, crowded, chipped, or cracked, they jump to the incorrect assumption that the person does not take care of himself. When someone has a well-groomed smile, not even a perfect smile, people do not jump to those conclusions and make snap judgments. Even if you cannot afford a perfect smile, small procedures can do a lot to improve your smile and change your life.

When a person is ashamed of the condition of her teeth/smile, she often doesn't smile or smiles without showing her teeth. This is often interpreted by the people she interacts with as the person being "unfriendly", and then, because people are inclined to mirror behavior, they tend to not smile or be friendly back. This can lead to isolation and reinforcement of the person feeling something's wrong with her—a vicious downward spiral. I've seen the personality and life of several of our patients completely change for the positive after having their smiles redone. One patient we'll call "June" visited us two years after a smile makeover and we initially didn't recognize her. She'd lost 50 pounds, was outgoing instead of mousy, and told us she'd gotten a new, better job with her newfound self-confidence!

At our office, we perform life-changing charity work—when we change someone's appearance, it changes her life forever. We participate in a program in our town called Hopeful Smiles, helping women who have overcome issues they have struggled with and turned their lives around. Even after getting their lives back together, they still have to look in the mirror and see how their choices destroyed their teeth. We replace missing teeth and perform minor cosmetic dental treatments to give them a better smile, so that they can get better jobs and not have to worry that their teeth are a distraction in their daily lives.

Since people are generally living longer, dentists are challenged with trying to keep patients' teeth healthy for 90+ years, something they have never had to do before. I look at my aging patients differently than I did 20 years ago, because I must predict what they may require in dental care in the future and plan how to help them maintain their oral health. Statistically speaking, the more teeth you have, the longer you live, because nutrition and digestion starts in the mouth. You must be able to chew good, crunchy, healthy food to maintain your health. If you enter your later stages of life with missing teeth, you end up with a bigger problem. Older patients take longer to heal from dental extractions, implants, or crowns. I work to set up my senior patients so they will have healthy dentition for the rest of their lives.

PRODUCTS TO IMPROVE YOUR SMILE KEEP GETTING BETTER

When someone asks me about the new developments in cosmetic dentistry, Invisalign® is the first thing that comes to my mind. Granted, it has been around for about 15 years and so is not completely new. However, the company is always developing new products and improvements on the original product to make it easier for the patient and the dentist to straighten teeth without wires, bands, and brackets. Invisalign® has impacted my practice a great deal because I can now use Invisalign® to straighten a patient's natural teeth to help create new smile. Before, I would have had to change a person's smile by drilling, removing teeth, and/or using porcelain. Now, with Invisalign® clear braces, many patients with otherwise beautiful teeth can get their teeth straightened into a beautiful smile without anyone knowing.

Invisalign® was first introduced to orthodontists for the sole purpose of making minor movement changes. With product improvements over the past 15 years, it is now the preferred treatment for certain kinds of crowding and alignment issues. For the past 10 years, it has been offered to general dentists to use with their patients. These tremendous improvements to the product and its constructive material, combined with new technology, have made Invisalign® a very important tool for cosmetic dentists. Today, when we use Invisalign®, we digitize the patient's mouth so that, with the computer, I can determine the best sequence of aligners or "trays" that will achieve the desired effect and alignment.

However, some things don't change. It still takes the same amount of time to move teeth with Invisalign® as it does with traditional metal braces. No matter how much you move the teeth, they can only be moved at a certain velocity or pace to maintain their health. If you move a tooth too fast, it responds negatively in a couple of ways. First, it will relapse—meaning it will quickly go back to its original position because the bone did not have time to heal and fill in where the tooth moved. Second, the roots will not respond correctly if we try to move the tooth too fast. In dentistry, quicker is not always better.

While Invisalign® takes the same amount of time to move your teeth, the advantage is that no one will notice Invisalign®; there are no wires, brackets, or bands. This is particularly important for professional adults who are in business or working in an industry where they command a certain level of respect. It may be difficult to maintain necessary levels of confidence when you have a mouth full of brackets and wires. Even though your colleagues may respect that you are taking steps to correct your smile, there is still a stigma associated with adults who have a mouth full of metal.

These differences have allowed me to become a more conservative dentist. Instead of cutting teeth and applying porcelain to improve a patient's smile, I can simply move his or her own teeth into perfect alignment. I still use porcelain in select cases. However, patients must deal with maintenance issues for the rest of their lives; whereas, if their teeth are aligned into the proper position, they will have a permanent beautiful smile. They can maintain the alignment by wearing a retainer at night, which is much easier than replacing the porcelain every 10 to 15 years. However, getting the teeth into alignment is often more important than using new applications, such as porcelain crowns or bridges versus Invisalign® plus a retainer, in the same way that aligning tires on your car is more important than the type of tire that you get. If you don't align the tires, they will fail sooner than they should. Teeth work on the same principle.

Anybody who wants to get his or her teeth straightened can be a candidate for Invisalign®. My patients have ranged in age from teenagers through senior citizens up to 81 years old. Invisalign® also creates a good foundation for other cosmetic dental work and products. I use it to bring teeth into proper alignment before installing crowns, bridges, or implants. As with home improvements, if you want to make an improvement to your house, you will ensure that the foundation is strong enough to support the additions or improvements. Your teeth are the same way. Before making improvements to your smile or oral health, make sure that you are starting with a good, strong foundation.

ADDITIONAL ADVANCEMENTS IN DENTISTRY WHICH RESULT IN A BEAUTIFUL SMILE MAKEOVER

Patients may not be aware of some of the newer technological tools, such as the digital mouth scanner. I use this in my office for taking impressions rather than having the patient bite down into the "goopy paste" that most people associate with dental impressions. We create a digital file and scan the patient's dentition (their teeth) into the computer to create a permanent record. From this digitized record or "complete scan", I can create crowns, bridges, dentures, and Invisalign® cases. Instead of the goopy paste, it is a permanent digital record of the patient's mouth. This increases the accuracy of many dental procedures that we perform.

The traditional way to make a crown is to drill the tooth, then use the goopy paste to make a negative impression of the tooth. That impression is sent to a laboratory where they will pour the material into the mold, fire the crown in an oven, and then return it to the dentist. There are all kinds of expansion and contraction factors involved throughout the process; I am amazed that these crowns fit by the time they are placed inside the patient's mouth. However, with a digital scanner, the image of the tooth is sent directly to the laboratory and a CAD/CAM machine fabricates the crown based on the digital scan. It is extremely accurate and much quicker, and it doesn't require a patient to sit for three to five minutes with a mouth full of goopy paste. The result is much better than we could ever achieve with the traditional way of creating crowns from molds.

Zirconia crowns do not get much attention, but I feel that they are a great advancement. Previously, when dentists needed to place a crown on a patient's tooth, we used a porcelain-fused-to-metal (PFM) crown. The metal was needed for its strength, but because no one wants metal displayed in their mouths, we would cover the metal with porcelain. About five years ago, Zirconia crowns were introduced and they have now replaced most of the PFM crowns for several reasons. One, there is always a chance of the porcelain shearing away from the metal because there are two layers of material. By contrast, Zirconia crowns are made from one layer of solid Zirconia. Two, people can always see a gray line around the gum line with PFM crowns because the metal shows below the porcelain. With Zirconia, metal is eliminated, so the beautiful smile has no gray lines. Three, Zirconia crowns are superior in color and hue compared to PFMs. The colors of the Zirconia crowns are every bit as natural-looking as their real teeth, and the translucency and vibrancy give spectacular results.

Lasers are another one of the advancements that I particularly like to use in my practice. When they think about cosmetic dentistry, most people think about changing their teeth. However, your gums are also a big part of your smile. You have probably seen people with "gummy smiles"—when they smile, you see too much of their gums. In my practice, we always try to achieve the perfect symmetry of a beautiful smile by adjusting the size, length, and shape of the teeth. When a patient has too much gum overlapping the tooth, I can use the laser to very gently contour the gum tissues and enhance the patient's smile—it's almost like trimming someone's cuticles. Plus, since there isn't bleeding or swelling with a laser, I can contour their gums and take impressions for veneers on the same visit, saving the patient an additional visit. I also use lasers to speed up the whitening process. After applying the bleaching solution to the patient's teeth, the laser activates the solution by speeding up the movement of the molecules. In one treatment, this accomplishes the same whitening that would normally take a week using the take-home trays.

The process of whitening teeth by using a form of hydrogen peroxide was actually discovered as a by-product of treating gum disease. Approximately 35 years ago, a periodontist named Dr. Keyes created a poultice of baking soda and hydrogen peroxide for patients to use in treating gum disease. Not only did patients' gums get better but their teeth also got whiter. Today, dentists use carbamide peroxide, and most of the commercial whitening products also use this as their basic ingredient. Early solutions were runny, inconvenient, and caused much more irritation than the solutions used today. Over the years, even the over-the-counter products have greatly improved.

The concentration level of the bleaching product is the difference between the in-office and over-the-counter whitening products, which have a much lower concentration of the bleaching agent than the products used in dental offices. As a patient, you would get the same results, but over-the-counter takes much longer than if you visit a dental office for a tooth whitening procedure. In addition to speed, another advantage of the in-office treatments includes the optional custom-made trays for your teeth. Our office scans the patient's mouth and fabricates a customized tray receptacle for the bleach, which is something you cannot get in an over-the-counter product. Even though the products sold in our office cost more when compared to over-the-counter products, there is much less waste when using a customized tray because the product has a stronger concentration.

I do recommend over-the-counter products for kids. Some children, as young as 10, may have yellowed teeth due to genetics. Their parents often ask me what they can do to whiten their child's teeth. If the child is in good health with healthy teeth, over-the-counter products are a good whitening option. However, with an adult, the longer your teeth have been discolored, the longer it will take to lighten them. Like bones in the desert sun, the longer they are exposed to the sun the whiter they become. Using the same principle, the more that you whiten teeth, the whiter they will become. As dentists, our responsibility is to do nothing that would harm the teeth or the health of our patients' mouths, so we use safe products. The negative consequence for our patients may be a little tooth sensitivity, but dentists can combat that sensitivity with topical products, Tylenol, and Advil. The sensitivity stops when the whitening stops; it is not a permanent side effect of the whitening process.

Missing teeth is one problem that I often see with my patients. However, my office has several ways to address this situation, from single tooth implants all the way up to a full set of prosthetic teeth. Traditionally, if a patient had a single missing tooth, dentists would use a three-unit bridge to replace the tooth. The two teeth on either side of the missing tooth would act as an anchor for the bridge holding the replacement tooth. However, this meant drilling away some of the enamel on each of the healthy teeth on either side of the gap to place the bridge. While three-unit bridges may still be the best solution in some cases, implants have given dentists a way to replace the missing tooth without drilling on the side teeth. A titanium post is surgically placed into the root location of the missing tooth, and then a crown is placed on top of the post.

Our office can also do what is called an "all-on-four" to replace an entire arch of teeth on the top, the bottom, or both top and bottom. The arch of teeth is permanently placed on the implants so that they are not removable like dentures. The implants are permanently screwed in place, which solves the common denture problem of "sliding". Once a year, the dentist removes the arch and checks underneath to ensure that the gums are healthy and everything still looks good. This is like the orthopedics of dentistry. As an orthopedist can manu- facture a replacement foot if you lose your foot in an accident, the dentist can create an arch of teeth if you are missing multiple teeth for any reason.

In the past, when a patient came into our office with a tooth weakened from a root canal and additional decay, we would need to further compromise the strength of the tooth by trying to repair it again. Now we can give the patient the option of replacing the tooth with an implant, to avoid the expense of re-

repairing the tooth with the risk that the procedure may fail. Many people assume the implant will be too expensive so they opt for trying to fix the new decay. In reality, the cost of an implant is about the same as having the canal re-treated, and making a new crown to be inserted over the tooth. For the number of people who have decay-prone teeth, constantly spending money to repair the same tooth is far more expensive and time-consuming than simply fixing the problem permanently with an implant. With the implant, there is nothing to decay or fail.

How To Find The Right Cosmetic Dentist

Other things change with time, such as the increasing need for people to find the right cosmetic dentist. Using the Internet, we can find reviews of almost everything, including dentists, with just a few clicks of the mouse. Dentists find that a well-reviewed practice is a successful practice because patients continually search for dentists who have received good reviews by previous and current patients. If a patient is moving and I cannot be her dentist any longer, I advise her to first look for a dentist who has a convenient location and then check the patient reviews.

Reviews are important. A dentist's great credentials do not necessarily mean he will be a good listener or that the patient's experience will be a good one. However, it's still important to check credentials as well as the dentist's continuing or advanced education. A good dentist will participate in continuing education courses to learn new techniques as well as keeping up-to-date on the latest advancements in cosmetic dentistry.

In addition to reviews, patients need to assess the skill of the dentist. The best method is to request to see the before and after pictures of previous patients. Most cosmetic dentists are proud to display before and after pictures; if the photos are posted on their website, you do not need to go into the office to see these pictures. Some dentists offer a list of patients who have had smile makeovers and are willing to share their experiences with other patients. Speaking to previous patients is an invaluable tool when you are looking for a cosmetic dentist.

However, do not forget that the dentist is only one part of the equation. Ask about the laboratory that the dentist uses to fabricate the porcelain crowns, veneers, and other dental implants. If the lab does not use quality materials or employ experienced technicians, the dentist can do beautiful work but the overall quality will be lacking due to poor-quality laboratory work. Most patients do not consider asking about the lab as an important element in choosing a cosmetic dentist, especially regarding the length of time that the dentist has used their particular lab. If a dentist hops around from lab to lab, it's a clue that there may not be problems with the lab but a problem with the dentist. Labs want to produce quality products and have success, not failure. If a dentist is exhibiting less than desirable impressions, scans, or techniques, the lab will tell the dentist that he or she needs to find another lab to do the work. Labs want to protect their reputation in the dental community, too.

In Dallas, there are several available dental laboratories but I have worked with the daVinci Laboratory in California for 20 years. I have an excellent relationship with the lab and the technicians who work there, which is important for my patients to receive the best products possible. For example, I can call the lab, and tell them that I have a client that is between x shade and y shade, so I need a little bit more of y color at the gum line but a little bit more of x color at the top of the tooth. I can create a customized, beautiful smile for my patient because I maintain good communication with a very good lab.

A unique combination of skill and talent makes a good dentist. However, the ability to communicate available options to the patient is a must. One of the nicest things about dentistry is that I do not ever have to choose from only one option to fix a problem. I have several tools and several ways to create the end product that best fits with my patient's current place in life. Maybe a procedure right now it is not financially feasible; however, we can often do a treatment now and plan on doing the more expensive treatment in 10 years. In dentistry, we can usually find an answer for all budget levels and all stages of life.

Some patients get concerned with the length of time that a smile makeover will last. While this is difficult to predict, the probability of success is greatly improved if a dentist begins with a strong, healthy foundation. For example, if a new patient comes into my office and tells me that this is his third broken crown, I take a step back to consider why this continues to happen. The crown failure may not be a problem with the crown or with the dentist, but possibly a problem with how the tooth is being hit when the patient bites down. If you do not take a step back to see why things are not successful, you are setting yourself up for failure. To avoid the problem in the future, I might recommend that the patient correct the alignment with Invisalign® before replacing the crown.

Another way to look at this would include the insurance company's perspective. Most insurance companies will not pay to replace a crown for at least five years after the crown was installed. Patients then assume that a crown should last at least five years; I agree, they should last much longer than that. If the crown breaks in four years, the patient panics at the dentist office because his insurance company will not pay to have the crown replaced. The dentist needs to look at the alignment, support, or other reasons for the failure of the crown. If the tooth decayed underneath the crown, the patient may be prone to decay, and it may be necessary to look at implants rather than replacing crowns. In an ideal world with every circumstance in its favor, including good alignment and the patient taking care of the crown, it should last a lifetime. However, the likelihood of the crown lasting depends a great deal on alignment. I always look at that first when considering a crown for one of my patients.

Unfortunately, dental insurance is very restrictive regarding specific items and how much they will pay for each service. Dental benefits plans usually have a maximum coverage of approximately $1,500 per year, which does not cover the cost for a single crown. As the purchasers of the policy, employers and the HR department determine the amount of annual coverage, the co-pay percentage, and what the dental insurance will and will not cover when purchasing dental policies for the employees. For example, most insurance policies view implants as "permanent restorations", falling under the category of major work, which is only covered at 50% of the total cost—the patient must pay the remaining balance. Research indicates that the implant is the most predictable, reliable, long-lasting replacement of a missing tooth. However, even though insurance companies know that implants are a much better option for patients who often have crowns replaced every few years, the insurance company will only cover the same percentage of the cost as they would for a crown. This situation is frustrating for dentists, because we want to practice according to what our patients need rather than what their insurance companies will cover, though we understand the importance of optimizing benefits as consumers. However, I am realistic about the situation and often find myself considering a treatment plan that the insurance company will cover that will also work for the patient.

ADVANCES IN TMJ TREATMENT

The frustrations of dental work are often outweighed by the advances we have made, such as in the treatment of TMJ. The Temporomandibular Joint (TMJ) is the joint where the jaw attaches to the skull. Because of the higher level of daily stress experienced by most people, they clench their jaws and grind their teeth. This produces broken teeth, worn dentition, and sore jaw joints. I follow the typical protocol and typical therapies for TMJ until they do not work any longer for my patients. If the patient has used the typical steps (i.e., a guard that is worn at night) but the pain has not subsided, a Botox application can relieve the pain in the major muscles that open and close the jaw.

Dentists began using Botox to relieve the pain and symptoms of TMJ after neurologists began using it to relieve migraines. Most migraine patients clench their jaws. When neurologists applied Botox for the migraine headaches, they noticed that the patients did not clench their jaws as much. Therefore, dentists began using the Botox application to treat TMJ. The injections can be life-changing for patients, because Botox relieves the pain associated with TMJ. One of my patients flew from Chicago to Dallas every three months for me to give him the

Botox injection. Literally, he would have a cab waiting downstairs for him to fly back home after his TMJ Botox shot at my office. I could have just found him someone in his area to do that, but he insisted.

For those who get that life-changing relief, the Botox gets applied every three months at first, with the intervals getting further and further apart. Muscle has memory, and if the memory is taken away from the muscle, they get atrophied, which brings back the symptoms. Patients don't commit to Botox every three months for the rest of their lives, but it does get people on their way toward healing, and it's a tremendous relief for the selected patients.

Having said that, the Botox procedure does not work for every TMJ patient, who must be screened carefully to ensure that the symptoms do not stem from another condition. I screen my patients thoroughly to ensure that they have followed the traditional treatments for TMJ before I recommend using Botox. In other words, if your symptoms are coming from an issue related to bony structures, such as the bone or the cartilage (between the skull and jaws) popping in and out with clicking noises, and the dentist has ruled out known muscle issues, then the Botox won't benefit you.

COMPOSITE VERSUS PORCELAIN

Another advance—which has relieved a different kind of pain—is seen in the difference between composite versus porcelain veneers. Composite is similar to a tooth-colored silly putty that dentists apply to the tooth. If a patient comes into the office and says, "I want bonding," that could cover a variety of treatments from the composite tooth-colored filling to bonding a veneer in place. Since I think that the public is confused about bonding, I will break down that idea, while first reviewing composite material.

Composite is a resin, a filler material that dentists use to fill in the back teeth. We use composite with our patients instead of using silver because composite is the same color as human teeth, and is bonded in place. A dentist can use composite in a lighter color to cover a person's tooth, called a "chairside veneer", making the tooth whiter without the need or the expense of using porcelain and a lab. Porcelain veneers are also bonded to the tooth just like composite material; however, they are made in a lab using a piece of porcelain and they are permanently bonded onto the tooth.

There are fewer options available for composite chairside veneers. For example, patients are limited to a certain number of colors by the dentist's skill in creating a veneer out of composite material and the composite is porous, so it will stain over time. The staining cannot be reversed with whitening products. Especially with a young person whose teeth are still changing and moving into place, dentists do not want to bond permanent veneers onto those teeth. With a broken or chipped tooth, dentists can use the composite resins to create a veneer until the patient is older. Later, composites can be replaced with permanent porcelain veneers. The downside to composite is that some dentists are better with hand skills while others are not as good at creating composite veneers in the office.

MY BEST ADVICE IS TO DO PREVENTIVE MAINTENANCE

My best advice is to do preventive maintenance—that is the key to a healthy, beautiful smile. The patient who does not come in on a regular basis for cleaning and exams will find that it is more costly in money and time to correct problems 10 or 15 years later, when they return to the dentist. Patients who avoid regular visits also experience more pain, because they generally require major treatments compared to those who come in for regular cleanings and minor treatments. With regular visits, a dentist can catch problems and correct them before they become major problems. It is staggering, the number of people who do not visit the dentist on a regular basis.

Consistent visits also give you a much better foundation to work with when dental problems are discovered. By catching problems early on, you do not need to compromise the tooth as much as when major problems must be fixed. The more dentists must compromise the tooth to correct a problem, the less of a chance you have that the work will last a long time. Preventive maintenance is the key. Also, insurance companies generally pay 100% for preventive dental care. Make sure that you get your cleanings and x-rays so that you can stay ahead of any problems.

(This content should be used for informational purposes only. It does not create a doctor-patient relationship with any reader and should not be construed as medical advice. If you need medical advice, please contact a doctor in your community who can assess the specifics of your situation.)

9

CONTINUING EDUCATION IS KEY TO FINDING THE RIGHT COSMETIC DENTIST TO GIVE YOU THE PERFECT SMILE

by Lois Kovalchick, D.D.S.

Continuing Education Is Key To Finding The Right
Cosmetic Dentist To Give You The Perfect Smile

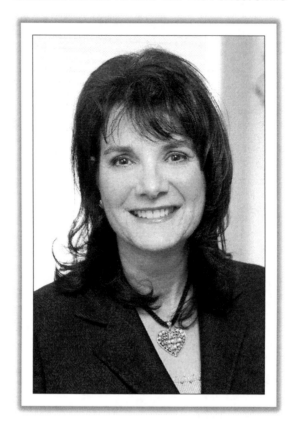

Lois Kovalchick, D.D.S.

Grosse Point Signature Smiles
Grosse Pointe Woods, Michigan
www.gpsmiles.com

Dr. Lois Kovalchick graduated with honors and received her Doctorate in Dental Surgery (DDS) from the University Of Detroit School Of Dentistry. She received a Bachelor of Science from the University of Detroit where she also received a degree as a Dental Hygienist. She completed the Comprehensive Dentistry Program at the Peter Dawson Academy and the Cosmetic Dentistry Program at the Louisiana State University School of Dentistry. She was an instructor at the University Of

Detroit School Of Dentistry for ten years. Dr. Kovalchick opened her practice in Grosse Pointe and has provided caring and exceptional dental care to her patients for over 25 years. Her concentration is in comprehensive dentistry with a special interest in cosmetic and implant dentistry.

For several consecutive years, Dr. Kovalchick was chosen as one of Metro Detroit's Top Dentists and featured in the Detroit Hour Magazine and Styleline Magazine. She is a recipient of the prestigious "Gold Metal" award presented by the American Academy of Cosmetic Dentists for her aesthetic dentistry. One of her endeavors is her participation with a charitable program named GBAS (Give Back a Smile). The charity is sponsored by the American Academy of Cosmetic Dentists and provides dental services to women who have been victims of domestic violence.

She has been an active member in her local dental association, the Detroit District Dental Society the Eastern division, holding official positions as Secretary, Treasurer, Vice President and President.

Dr. Kovalchick maintains an active membership in the American Dental Association and the Michigan Dental Association. She is also a member of the American Academy of Cosmetic Dentistry.

CONTINUING EDUCATION IS KEY TO FINDING THE RIGHT COSMETIC DENTIST TO GIVE YOU THE PERFECT SMILE

When choosing a cosmetic dentist, I believe it is important for the dentist to have received additional training by attending continuing education programs that address comprehensive dental care. What I mean by comprehensive dental care is dental care that not only "looks good" but "functions" as well. This is extremely important because patients who want cosmetic dental procedures to enhance their smile often may have significant underlying dental problems that are contributing to their situation. For example, a patient may present with "smaller teeth" because they have been worn down by a functional issue that is destroying the teeth and yet he (or she) wants his teeth to look like they used to. The "functional" problem needs to be evaluated and possibly treated in con-junction with the patient's aesthetic desires. Cosmetic dentistry ranges from simply wanting whiter teeth to the need for a team approach involving a general dentist to include specialist(s) to achieve desirable results. As a dentist who provides cosmetic dentistry, one needs to be able to address both of these components. To do this, the dentist must have a background in "functional dentistry" as well as cosmetic procedures and therefore has the knowledge and capabilities to practice "functional cosmetic dentistry." There are many programs available for dentists who want to expand their practice and gain more experience in this area. In my opinion, you want a dentist who is committed pursuing this level of excellence.

For example, I have completed several cosmetic courses at LSU that included lectures, hands-on experience, and homework involved with completing and submitting projects. I also completed the Dawson Program which places a heavy emphasis on "functional dentistry". When you add up all of the time I put into these programs and other training, it would total several months of training. This type of training is very different from taking a one-day course that discusses cosmetic dentistry. There are several institutes and universities which have multi-level programs that teach comprehensive dental care with an emphasis on cosmetics such as the Pankey, the Dawson, and the Spear Institutes, just to mention a few. A dentist is able to master each level as he or she progresses through the program. If I were searching for a cosmetic dentist, I would be looking on the walls in the practice to see what type of training the dentist has accomplished and in what areas of dentistry. I would strongly recommend that you evaluate the dentists' work by viewing before and after photographs of their patients who have completed cosmetic procedures and by reading testimonials from patients who have had cosmetic dental care.

Also, consider what professional groups or associations the dentist is active in or a member of when researching a cosmetic dentist. For example, I am a member of the Seattle Study Club. It is a national dental organization comprised of general dentists and specialists geared to the implementation of comprehensive dental care. We have structured meetings as a group that include completing modules in continuing education. But, what I really like is that it provides us the opportunity as a group to act as a "think tank", where we can discuss the treatment of patients that need additional attention of a specialist(s) as well as a general dentist in order to achieve a great outcome when having cosmetic dentistry. Also, I am a member of the American

Academy of Cosmetic Dentistry (AACD). A dentist that is a member of the AACD or other associations has a great opportunity to take continuing education courses. Affiliation with professional group(s) and a passion for continuing education are good indicators that the dentist is staying current and abreast of the rapid advancements occurring in dentistry

MY PHILOSOPHY IS "CONSERVATIVE DENTISTRY"

When I began my career as a dentist, there was no term for what is now called minimally invasive dentistry. I previously coined the term "conservative dentistry" when I described my philosophy to my patients as a dental practitioner. So what is my definition of conservative dentistry? It is the preservation of the ENAMEL of the tooth. I believe that the main benefit for the patient in utilizing this approach is that you are not compromising or weakening the tooth by unnecessarily removing the enamel. Once the enamel of the tooth is removed, it is irreversible. Therefore, you want to preserve as much of it as possible to keep the integrity of the tooth. Conservative Dentistry has been the core principle of my practice, the focus of my continuing education, and my philosophy as a dentist.

My desire to protect and preserve the enamel on the teeth developed about 20 years ago when I implemented air abrasion technology into my practice. I did this because I had many children as patients for whom I recommended sealants on their permanent back teeth. In order for the sealant to stay on the tooth and not pop off, you must begin with a very clean tooth. By using air abrasion technology to clean the teeth prior to applying the sealant, I found that the sealant stayed in place. A sealant is a preventative procedure that protects the tooth from getting cavities. It works like applying a clear-coat on a vehicle in order to protect the surface paint from the outside elements. A sealant gives you that extra layer of protection.

But, I sometimes discovered when I used the air abrasion technology to clean out the grooves on the top of the tooth, I would reveal a cavity that was not noticeable on an x-ray and was not visible during a clinical exam. The cavity was minimal and I was able to remove the decay using the air abrasion technology and restore the tooth with a simple white filling. Therefore, I began to perform "conservative fillings" for these children and not waiting for the cavity to become bigger, requiring numbing of the child's tooth, using the drill to remove the cavity, and the placement of a silver filling which was traditionally done at that time. I concluded that I was doing a great service for these children and they have grown up in my practice having either no cavities or having minimal fillings and therefore have natural looking teeth. This has to be one of the most fulfilling things I have experienced as a practicing dentist. Over all, this was my epiphany and it made me think in a different way. I wanted to find ways to preserve the enamel on all of my patients' teeth.

With traditional dentistry, the history of treating cavities is to remove the decay by drilling out the cavities and filling them with silver. As time goes by, the tooth can develop new decay or the filling/restoration breaks down; so the dentist removes the filling and the decay with the drill and now the restoration is larger. Years later, the cusp of the tooth breaks off and then the tooth requires a crown to protect the remaining tooth structure. Instead of going through this historical process, I became committed to being proactive and I believe the best method of treatment is to apply sealants to the permanent back teeth and treat cavities in their earliest stage and, as a result, maintain the integrity of the enamel on the tooth. This is how I clinically achieved a generation of patients with no cavities and natural looking teeth.

As I continued on my path of "conservative dentistry", I began to take extensive training courses in how to provide different types of restorations for teeth that required less removal of the enamel. This method of treatment included restorations known as ceramic inlays, onlays, veneers, and three-quarter crowns which did not require the more aggressive removal of the enamel on the tooth as required when restoring teeth with full coverage crowns. Then I began doing what I call "designer preparations". I would design laboratory-made restorations that enabled me to prepare the tooth in such a way as to preserve as much enamel as possible. As I continued to learn more about cosmetic dentistry, I started combining these types of restorations while planning my patients' treatments which allowed for the preservation of their enamel. For example, instead of delivering two crowns, I might do a crown on one tooth and a restoration on the other tooth, such as an onlay (partial crown), that requires less enamel to be removed. In my opinion, a crown should be the last resort when restoring a tooth.

THE BEST WAY TO MOVE TEETH

I am a big believer that it is always better to have teeth in their proper position and alignment before cosmetic dentistry is initiated. For example, if you have two front teeth that are severely crisscrossed, it is always better to uncross them through orthodontic movement with braces than to attempt to change the appearance of the teeth through new restorations alone. Taking a short-cut and restoring the teeth without their proper position can result in the bone and gums being compromised and thereby creating areas that are hard to keep clean or areas that are bulky and lead to gum irritation. It is always better to move teeth into proper alignment through orthodontics rather than through restorations.

I am often asked about Invisalign® for moving crooked teeth. Invisalign® is appealing to patients because they do not have the wires and brackets that you have with traditional braces. Patients are very receptive of Invisalign® as an orthodontic treatment and may obtain good results. However, not every patient is a candidate for Invisalign®. Sometimes a patient has a more complex situation where traditional orthodontics would be better for his or her circumstance. If a patient presents with a skeletal discrepancy or has a history of jaw pain or other functional issues, it may be better for the patient to have traditional orthodontic treatment.

Every technique or method of treatment has it parameters. Therefore, the dentist should be familiar with several techniques so he or she can utilize the one that works best or more appropriately for the patient. For example, if you have a sports car, you may very well want to drive 70 mph down the interstate, but you would not take the same vehicle off-roading, much less do 70 mph when off-roading. There are certain methods for treating certain conditions just as there are certain tools for certain jobs. Working within the parameters for and selecting the right method is essential for a successful outcome.

YOU MUST LOOK AT THE WHOLE PICTURE...
EVERY PICTURE TELLS A STORY

When performing and delivering successful cosmetic dentistry, one must look at the whole picture. It is all about the patient. Understanding the patients' dental needs and determining how you can guide and help them achieve what they are looking for during the planning process of the cosmetic treatment is a big part of the picture. A dentist must have good "people skills" as well as technical skills to be successful in fulfilling the patient's expectations. In addition, it is equally important to have a great staff and a clean and comfortable office setting. Being successful is really about being well-rounded.

I connect with my patients by having openly honest and relaxed conversations. I look at them eye-to-eye and sincerely ask, "What is it that you are looking for and how can we help you get what you desire?" I often start this by taking photographs of the patients and, together, we analyze their smiles. Also, I allow them to take the photographs home with them so that they can think over what we have discussed. I advise them to take their time and study their pictures and jot down some notes of what they like and what they don't like. By doing this exercise, I get a better idea of where to start my treatment planning based on the patient's desires.

For example: The patient might come back and say, "You know what? My teeth are crooked." Okay, we have a starting point and we can begin by talking about straightening his teeth either with Invisalign® or by braces/orthodontics. Or she says, "I like my smile but my teeth are not as white as I would like them to be." Alright, let's determine if you are a candidate for having your teeth whitened. As you can see this gives me a place to start to address their cosmetic concerns.

The reason I prefer to use a photograph of the patient is simple: I am trying to make it more individualized, practical, and, therefore, real for the patient. I have had patients come into my practice with a magazine picture of a model that they would like to look like. Even though I do appreciate the input and can use it as a guideline or reference, I prefer to use the patient's photograph because it allows me to customize the smile. Also, I am not treating that model, I am treating my patient. It's similar to taking picture of a model with gorgeous hair to your hairdresser and asking her to recreate the exact same look. She may first tell you that you can't achieve the same color of hair or you do not have the kind of hair to duplicate the results you expect. Therefore, by using photographs of the patients themselves, I have a better foundation for addressing their issues and giving them some parameters for more realistic expectations.

When I evaluate a patient seeking cosmetic dentistry, I first look at the general health of the mouth to determine if there is any disease present, such as cavities or gum infections. Then I evaluate for signs of functional problems and aesthetic issues. From there, I take a set of radiographs (x-rays), several photographs of the patient and fabricate a set of models of the teeth and gums to be used for a "functional cosmetic analysis". During the planning process for comprehensive dental treatment I am looking at form, function, and what looks good in general. A benefit of being a member of a study group is that we evaluate cases together that may need additional treatment by a specialist along with development of a methodology and guidelines for comprehensive dental treatment. I have developed my own formula when I evaluate for dental disease, functional issues, and aesthetic issues. Some of these guidelines can be three or four pages in length; I have an entire check-off sheet that I use when I meet with a patient. I look at the photographs of the patient, I look at the models, and I listen to what the patient is telling me that he or she desires. I go through the formula—which I have developed based on my training, education, and experience—to determine the appropriate treatment. I use my plan to make a prototype and a duplicate set of models to ensure that what I have planned can be done. Before I do any cosmetic makeover, I know where I am headed.

The patient is informed about the recommended procedures to be used, the estimated timetable, what the anticipated results are, and the cost. The patient can evaluate the prototype to see how he or she likes it before we begin treatment. Also, I like to study the case along with the patient and, if needed, have the opportunity to make changes, even minor refinements, before proceeding. Whenever compromises are made, that is discussed and dealt with up front. Patients appreciate it when you commit the time and give this type of attention regarding their treatment. It builds a relationship between the dentist and the patient. The patient is more comfortable, committed, and excited to begin treatment.

After patients have completed cosmetic dentistry I have found that they smile more—perhaps because they feel more confident in their appearance. If you are more confident when you smile and portray a friendly, happy attitude, it can't help but change your life. For instance, I play this silly game which I call the "Smile Game" while I am jogging. Sometimes I will smile at people as we pass each other and, like a universal language, they smile back at me. Other times, when I cross path with someone,

I wait to see if the other person will smile first and many times the chance of smiling first is missed; therefore I often have to initiate with a smile first to have a person reciprocate. What's interesting is that I have noticed that those to whom I have first initiated a smile, will now be the first to smile at me without hesitation. A smile has unbelievable power. If you are holding back your smile, then you are cutting yourself off from a lot of experiences in life that are out there waiting for you. People who have cosmetic work done are more likely to show it off and be more relaxed because they no longer feel self-conscious about their smiles anymore. In a nutshell, I believe that cosmetic dentistry improves my patients' lives.

The best dentistry is the minimum amount of dentistry needed to accomplish the goal and goes back to the minimal invasiveness approach. If a person does not like his or her teeth because they are crooked but are otherwise healthy and look good, it is better for that person to simply straighten the teeth. If a person has dark teeth and desires them to be whiter, it is better just to whiten the teeth rather than prepping the teeth to do veneers. With regard to whitening teeth, we have many different options from which to choose.

WHITENING YOUR SMILE

In my practice, we have three or four different ways we can enhance one's smile by whitening the teeth. It all depends on how light the patient desires the teeth to be and how committed or compliant he or she is during the whitening process. For example, some patients prefer to wear custom trays filled with a whitening product that requires two to four weeks to lighten their teeth. Others choose to have their teeth whitened in a couple of hours which can be done as an in-office procedure. And some just want the maximum effect and we can do what I call a "whitening booster" in the office in combination with products to use at home. It all depends on how dark the teeth are and what the patient is willing to do to achieve the results he or she desires.

Of course, there are economic considerations. If a patient is looking for a very inexpensive way to whiten her teeth, she may try the over-the-counter whitening products. They usually have limited results but they are great for some circumstances. For example, a teenager who wants to have whiter teeth for the upcoming high school prom.

On the other hand, as time goes by, our teeth are exposed to certain drinks, such as cola, red wine, coffee, and tea, and also some foods that can stain our teeth. Our teeth become stained from the repeated consumption of such drinks and foods. Therefore, professional whitening is often best to aid in reducing these stains and achieving the desired results.

One factor that deters patients from having their teeth whitened is a fear or a previous history of sensitive teeth. However, the products we have today are much better and we have ways to prevent and deal with sensitivity issues throughout the professional whitening process.

GUM LIFTS

The gum tissue surrounding the teeth has an important role and greatly contributes to the success and final results of having of cosmetic dentistry. The gum tissue serves as the background for displaying the teeth in one's smile. If there is a visual distraction in the background, such as uneven gum tissue, it will be noticeable in your overall appearance. Therefore, it is important to have symmetry involving the gum tissue in order to achieve a pleasing smile. Sometimes, a patient will display too much gum tissue or not show enough tooth structure for his or her smile. These may be instances where a gum lift is recommended. In order to get the result that the patient desires, we must address this in addition to any other cosmetic treatment that we have planned.

I sometimes sense patients have a nervous reaction when mentioning gum lifts because they perceive their aesthetic problem is related only to having bad teeth and therefore are primarily focused on "fixing their teeth". This is where the diagnostic work-up is effective. In most cases, by using a prototype/mock-up to illustrate what the end result will look like when incorporating a gum lift as part of the treatment plan, they will agree to the recommended treatment to achieve a more pleasing result. If the patient can visualize that one tooth is going to look a lot longer than the other teeth, it is easier to make the right decision to correct the aesthetic problem.

Also, the diagnostic workup and fabrication of a mock-up are helpful in determining if we are able to correct the gum issues by using a laser or if a surgical gum lift is required. We want to know this up front and integrate this as part of the full plan. In some cases, a gum lift can be accomplished with the use of a laser to remove excess gum tissue and make minor corrections. Many times, I am able to use the laser to simply do a few touchups. The advantage of using a laser is that it is a less invasive procedure with a faster healing response. However, there are cases where a patient may need a surgical gum lift to correct the aesthetic problems.

BONDING & CONTOURING FOR A BEAUTIFUL SMILE

Another question I am often asked is "Can you bond my teeth and make them look better?" In my practice, I have treated several patients with resin bonded restorations for aesthetic improvements. I favor bonded restorations for a lot of reasons. Primarily, it preserves more enamel in comparison to other types of restorations and, for the most part, it is a reversible procedure. Another reason I especially like them is that they are repairable. If you are active in playing sports you may be more subjected to injuries including trauma to your teeth. If chipping or fracturing occurs, bonded restorations can be repaired more easily, unlike porcelain restorations. Also, for younger patients whose teeth may not be fully erupted and will require future touch-ups or retreatment as the patient is growing; bonded restorations are the way to go. I can easily adjust and contour the tooth by adding resins to it. Typically, I prefer doing resin bonded restorations for younger patients and those who have never had any previous type of cosmetic treatments—that is, of course, if the patient is a candidate.

The downside to resin bonded restorations is that it does not allow for a big change in the color of your teeth. So if you are seeking a huge change in the color of your teeth, resin bonding is probably not your best option. However, they work really well for a patient who wants to close spaces between teeth or increase the size of an underdeveloped or a small tooth such as a peg lateral, if space is not limited. The other concern is that they are more prone to staining and wear compared to other types of cosmetic restorations. For the most part, adult patients who are looking for a whiter smile to include better shape and sizes to their teeth and have had a lot of previous fillings in their front teeth may consider other types of cosmetic procedures rather than "bonding".

TECHNOLOGY'S LINK TO CONTINUING EDUCATION

The real story is, the more knowledge a dentist has obtained and the mastering of different techniques the more he or she can offer and deliver cosmetic solutions to their patients. It is similar to what that old adage says, "If the only tool you have is a hammer, everything looks like a nail." On the other hand, with knowledge in the various types of treatment in cosmetic dentistry—such as whitening, bonding, veneers, partial crowns and gum lifts, just to name a few—the dentist can offer and provide the best service for that patient's individual situation.

The use of technology in dentistry is leading to drastic advancements and changes in the delivery of services to patients as it is in all areas of the medical field. For example, we can now use a digital scanner in the fabrication of restorations rather than taking an impression and making molds of teeth. We can scan the tooth with a digital scanner and are able to send the image to the lab and the lab, thereby, produces the restoration. Also, there is CAD/CAM technology that allows the dentist to fabricate the restoration right in the office. It is very precise and fast, meaning there is less time involved in delivering the final restoration. As the technology continues to evolve and become more affordable, I believe more dentists will adopt the newer technology and acquire the knowledge to implement it in the practice. This is where the learning continuum is so important because it allows the dentist to provide the best service. You must be exposed to all the various levels of expertise and mastering the art.

IT'S TIME TO DO SOMETHING FOR YOURSELF

Many times, I have patients in my practice who have spent a great deal of their lives taking care of others and now they want to do something for themselves. I often hear, "It's MY time now and I want to do something to make myself look better and feel better about my appearance." This is where we can begin to explore options. It could simply be whitening their teeth and that is good enough for them to feel great about their smiles. Often, I can make subtle changes that make a huge difference. However, it could be a situation where we need to do extensive dental treatment to correct functional issues tied in with cosmetic concerns. In any case, I hesitate to make recommendations until we research your options for what can be done to freshen up your smile.

For the most part, when patients are seeking help to improve their smiles, they want the end results to look natural. We have all seen cosmetic dentistry that has been taken to the extreme and looks phony; and upon interacting with them, the only thing that grabs your attention are the six over-the-top, super-white porcelain veneers that don't seem to "fit". I often joke with my patients by saying, "When you enter the room, you don't want your teeth to enter before you do." So no one really wants to look like she has had "work done", but she wants to look fresh. That is the big difference between looking at someone who has had cosmetic dentistry done and thinking to yourself, "WOW, she has a gorgeous smile!" and looking at someone and asking yourself, "When did she get those veneers?"

I believe this is where I can help my patients. As a dentist, I do not know what it will take to freshen up a person's smile until we spend the time together. If you were to come to my office with this frame of mind, we would sit down together, review your options for enhancing your smile, and make a plan with which you are comfortable and that accomplishes your goal.

(This content should be used for informational purposes only. It does not create a doctor-patient relationship with any reader and should not be construed as medical advice. If you need medical advice, please contact a doctor in your community who can assess the specifics of your situation.)

10

A BEAUTIFUL SMILE WILL FOREVER CHANGE YOUR LIFE!

by Ryan F. Ziegler, D.M.D.

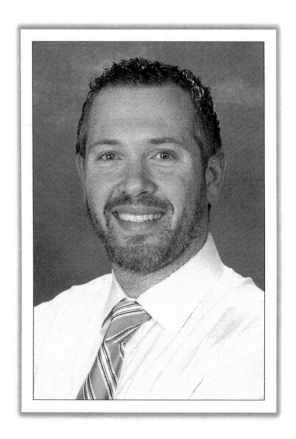

Ryan F. Ziegler, D.M.D.
Miami Center for Cosmetic and Implant Dentistry
Miami, Florida
www.miamicosmeticdentalcare.com

Dr. Ryan F. Ziegler has treated thousands of happy patients and he is known as a leading cosmetic dentist in Miami and South Florida.

Dr. Ziegler practices at the Miami Center for Cosmetic and Implant Dentistry offering Brite Smile teeth whitening, dental implants, porcelain veneers, dentures, teeth-in-a-day, sedation dentistry, emergency dentistry and more. He is highly-trained in all types of cosmetic dentistry procedures, including tooth whitening, bridges, crowns, and veneers. As part of his comprehensive approach to dentistry, Dr. Ziegler works with your schedule to help ensure that you can receive the dental assistance that you need to have the smile that you want. Dr. Ziegler also works to make your cosmetic dentistry procedures affordable.

Dr. Ziegler uses his education and experience to help patients achieve the smile that they have dreamed of for so long. His passion for his patients comes through in the way that he invests the time necessary to learn about his patients and their desires.

A BEAUTIFUL SMILE WILL
FOREVER CHANGE YOUR LIFE!

Over the years, many of my patients at the Miami Center for Cosmetic and Implant Dentistry have expressed their thoughts on the importance of an attractive smile, and many more patients desire an attractive smile even if they don't bring it up in conversation or think they may not be able to afford it. It is indisputable that the importance and value of an attractive smile is immeasurable. It falls into categories, such as a "first date". When you meet that special someone, you do not want to feel the need to hide your smile or be self-conscious about first impressions. An attractive smile is one of the first things that people notice about us. It is important for succeeding at work and getting the job of your dreams. It helps you make new friends and be more socially active. In our current society, people are more likely to accept someone with a nice smile. They often believe that having bad teeth is indicative of bad personal hygiene, low social status, or even lack of intelligence. Smiles are important, especially in the social arena. Your smile is one of the very first things that a person will notice about you, and bad teeth can overshadow the rest of your appearance, from your pretty eyes to your nice hair. It's unfortunate but true that having a nice smile (versus an unattractive smile) tremendously influences one's self-esteem. In today's world, what accentuates the negative impact of an unattractive smile is that achieving a remarkable "before and after result" is often easily and quickly attainable.

Most of my patients already know the main problem with their smile, but they often overlook a few other aspects that need enhancing. If I only fixed the things that my patients initially wanted to be changed, the end result would often be unsatisfactory. My job is to review everything with them so that they see the big picture, which also helps me to see what the patient wants to achieve. Some patients want absolute perfection while others just want an improvement. Also, some patients have several things cosmetically wrong with their teeth but just want one thing fixed. While I ultimately need to give my patients what they want (it's the patient's mouth, not mine), at the same time, I need to do what is best for them and give my best guidance.

What is extremely important for the patient to understand is that cosmetic dentistry requires an artistic acumen and talent that separates this facet of dentistry from all other categories of dental treatment. I believe a true cosmetic dentist must be an artist and have a unique appreciation of the many components that contribute to attaining the desired state of perfection. One may argue that perfection is unattainable. However I suggest that striving towards a goal of perfection will ultimately yield results well beyond the patient's expectations.

My initial goal is to create an immediate cosmetic change on the very first visit. It is a regular and common occurrence for my patient to leave after the first visit with a beautiful smile. This is achieved by the fabrication of temporary crowns or veneers that create an extreme improvement of the patient's initial smile. It is extremely gratifying to see the metamorphosis my patient goes through after just a few hours of treatment. Although we give the patients initial before and after photos prior to beginning treatment, most find it hard to believe that they are really going to be the recipients of that incredible change they've always dreamed of having. My greatest personal reward is the exuberance my patients express when they see their end results. The myriad of emotions they express on that final day when they look into the mirror is priceless. To think that I have been so blessed to have been the beneficiary of this experience from thousands of patients over the years is a true gift for me.

During the first evaluation, I ask the patient to open his or her mouth and smile for me. I then step back a few feet to assess the mouth the way that another person would look at him or her on a casual basis. Without focusing on an individual tooth, I get a broad sense of his or her smile line. Are the teeth long or short, narrow or wide? Do the teeth slant off to one side or dip down? This gives me a sense of which route to take when developing a plan for a smile makeover. It may involve straightening the teeth with Invisalign®, following a simple re-contouring and bonding route, or applying porcelain techniques. As I continue to take a closer look, I may determine that the patient has significant tooth damage (worn, discolored, or fractured) or that an asymmetrical gum line is adding to his or her dental problems.

During the consultation, I use "before and after" photos of my prior cases. Patients can look through them, make sure that they view the end results of a variety of my previous makeovers, and appreciate the type of transformations that can be made in the mouth. One of my favorite things to mention to patients during a consultation is the fact that, unlike any other cosmetic procedure, cosmetic dentistry allows patients to see the end result before it is brought to completion. This allows the patient to give final approval for an end result that lives up to expectations and is exactly what is wanted. In some cases, I use study models so that patients can get a mock-up of their own mouths to use in the process of designing customized cosmetic procedures.

With prototypes, patients can see how their new smile will appear in their mouth before we apply the permanent produce. A patient can give the green light and say, "Doc, I'm thrilled with what I see. Let's finish it off." We can then permanently bond the veneers or crowns to the teeth. However, a patient may say, "I really like everything I'm seeing except one or two aspects. Can this be changed? Can the veneer be made wider or longer?" As always, any aspect of the case can be changed. Patients return for a subsequent appointment to see the change. If that is acceptable, we place it in the mouth for a final bonding or cementation. Patients appreciate the fact that they get to approve their cosmetic end result before it is completed in the mouth. That is why I never have a patient leave unhappy: in the end, everyone is always thrilled.

Our patients are usually overwhelmed when they see themselves for the first time after we finish the work. When I hand the patient a mirror, he or she is overjoyed, seeing a new smile for the first time. Words cannot describe the feeling I get, seeing my patients overcome with joy and tears, seeing themselves as they always dreamed they should look. Countless patients have come back to tell me that they wished they had "done this sooner."

A patient in her 50s came to see me about a smile makeover. I did a full mouth upper and lower arch porcelain veneer reconstruction. She was ecstatic with the results and said it was the best thing she had ever done. Recently, she came into my office and told me that her only problem is that her cheeks hurt from smiling so much. She found herself walking past windows and mirrors smiling at herself all the time. For years prior to her treatment, she had to cover her mouth every time she smiled because she was so self-conscious about her teeth, and now she has self-confidence when talking with people. During one of her regular six-month cleanings, she started crying with gratitude and appreciation for what we had done for her.

In my office, for years I typically saw more women than men who want a smile makeover. However, there's been a significant increase in the number of men wanting aesthetic dental treatment. Often, I see younger men in their 20s to 40s who are starting careers, seeking a different job, or looking for new relationships. However, in recent years, we've experienced a noticeable increase in baby boomers and seniors seeking cosmetic improvements with their smiles. Ultimately, most people are looking to elevate their self-esteem and cosmetic dentistry affords the solution.

For example, one patient came to my office because he felt uncomfortable applying for jobs with his current smile. This 42-year-old gentleman was unhappy, had low self-esteem, and was very self-conscious. He always had felt that people were staring at his mouth. After his smile makeover, he had the courage to reapply for a sales job that he wanted and had been turned down for the previous year. He told me, "Dr. Ziegler, the same person that interviewed me a year earlier remembered me and at the end of the interview actually commented about my infectious smile. I was shocked we he told me that, but the end result was that I got the job!" My patient told me that he has turned into a real extrovert and has much more self-confidence when initially meeting people. He gives full credit to his new smile for his personality-altering transformation and I am the recipient of his thanks and appreciation. How much better does it get! The following week, two of his coworkers came to see me and began cosmetic treatment.

An additional advantage that we offer patients at the Miami Center for Cosmetic and Implant Dentistry is the wide scope of dental implant treatment we provide. Often, my patients' treatment involves not only cosmetic treatment with porcelain veneers and crowns, but dental implants as well. In our office, I work in tandem with Dr. Gonzalo Barrantes, whose focus is on every aspect of implant dentistry and all the latest "state of the art" implant procedures. The end result is that, together, in a short period of time, we can achieve results in our single office location that are truly spectacular. There are some patients whose teeth are not salvageable due to extensive decay or advanced periodontal disease. They simply are not candidates for cosmetic dentistry utilizing some or all of their natural teeth. In these cases, rather than subjecting a patient in this category to treatment and an expense which is doomed to failure, working together, we are able to achieve predictable, stable, and beautiful long term results utilizing dental implants. Patients in this category, who initially arrive in our office downtrodden and depressed, leave feeling they have a new lease on life.

Outside of the office, I personally enjoy playing piano, basketball, traveling—and most importantly, my family. Inside the office, my reward is giving patients a reason to smile again. This may be a cliché statement but it is true all the same. Of course I enjoy changing a patient's perception of dentistry, but mostly, I enjoy the new sense of confidence that patients receive with their smile makeovers. I feel that I am a cosmetic architect for the mouth. As a member of the American Dental Association, Florida Dental Association, South Florida Dental Association, American Academy of Cosmetic Dentistry, and others, I keep up-to-date on all of the latest advancements in cosmetic dentistry. Dentistry is my passion and helping people is my purpose.

I tell my patients that there are six ways to improve the appearance of their smile using cosmetic dentistry: teeth whitening, bonding, porcelain veneers, porcelain crowns, Invisalign®, and gum reshaping (aka "gingival reshaping"). The route that I choose to help a patient improve their smile will depend on that specific patient.

TEETH WHITENING

For teeth whitening, there are three basic methods. The least expensive method includes over-the-counter products sold at local drugstores. These products do achieve some results for patients, though not to the level of the other two options. Custom trays, the middle-of-the-road route, are made by the dentist to perfectly fit the mouth and teeth so the whitening gel can adapt to the front surface of the teeth. This will give the patient a better result than the over-the-counter products. The simplest whitening method is more costly but far more effective and less time consuming: a professional in-office whitening procedure. This short procedure is done during one appointment in the dentist's office. A patient can walk in and leave after two hours with much whiter teeth.

Before a patient decides on a whitening strategy, he (or she) should discuss all procedures with a dentist in order to determine if he is a good candidate for teeth whitening. For instance, if you have heavily stained teeth, you cannot expect exceptional results. If you have old dental work, bondings, or porcelain, this rules out a good candidacy for teeth whitening since the artificial material will not whiten along with your enamel. If a tooth has intrinsic staining—meaning it has a darker core from internal stains—this isn't good for whitening because the darker core gives the tooth a grayish hue. Generally, that tooth will not whiten well.

BONDING

Bonding has been used for a long time and serves a purpose, though it has a shorter life expectancy compared to porcelain treatments. Generally, bonding gives a less optimal cosmetic outcome because the bonding material itself does not have the natural translucence of a quality porcelain product. Bonding is typically used for more minor corrective needs.

In some instances, improving one's smile is a very simple process that can be done with contouring and bonding (both go hand-in-hand) without needing to go to the length of orthodontics or even Invisalign® and veneers. Good candidates for contouring and bonding are patients with small problems in one or a few teeth. The contouring aspect involves carefully shaping the existing tooth by removing small amounts of the tooth around the edges. This contouring gives the patient a more even smile. It also gets rid of the chipped and worn appearance of the teeth.

For patients with pronounced canines (the "vampire" appearance), contouring is ideal. Some of my patients had consulted other dentists before coming to my office, and those dentists were ready to do a full set of porcelain veneers. I told them, "Wait, I'm going to make you very happy. Within a half hour, I can transform your smile simply and quickly and you'll spend a fraction of the cost of veneers." With a conservative contouring and bonding application, the patients walk out within one hour, thrilled with the end result and the fact that I had just saved them from unnecessarily spending a bunch of money to improve their smile.

The cost of cosmetic dentistry can vary widely. Generally, but not always, the cost associated with cosmetic dentistry depends on several factors. For example, porcelain material is more expensive than bonding material. Therefore, a patient will pay more for porcelain veneers than for contouring and bonding. The cost of cosmetic dentistry also depends on the dentist's skill level, the location of the dentist's practice, the techniques, and the dentist's laboratory.

The cost of the cosmetic work also depends on the level of work that must be performed in order to accomplish the patient's goal. Some patients may not be suitable candidates for contouring and bonding, so veneers would be the better option. The cost of the cosmetic work greatly depends on the type of work being performed and the amount of work involved in correcting other issues. Since each patient's situation is different, one patient cannot base the cost of his cosmetic work on another patient's cost.

Unfortunately, most dental insurance policies do not cover cosmetic dentistry, with a few exceptions. For example, when the main purpose of cosmetic dentistry is to repair a structural problem that could affect the oral health, dental insurance would cover the cost of cosmetic dentistry. However, patients should not get their hopes up about insurance coverage. Since cosmetic dentistry can become expensive, I work with third-party financing in my office. It allows patients to get the beautiful smile they want without waiting years to save up the money. Third-party financing can make cosmetic dentistry affordable for patients.

PORCELAIN VENEERS

Veneers can transform a smile in as few as two dental visits. Veneers drastically change the appearance of an individual's smile by altering the color, shape, size, and overall appearance of the teeth. Some veneer cases are done with as few as two veneers while other cases may involve 20 veneers. While I like to guide patients into the best possible outcome, I do offer different options and quantities of veneers, thoroughly explaining the end results that can be achieved based on those options.

A porcelain veneer is a semi-translucent shell that is handcrafted from durable porcelain, custom shaded, and then permanently bonded to the tooth. Porcelain veneers involve some anesthetic because the teeth are mildly reshaped to allow room for the porcelain laminate to be adhered and bonded to the tooth. They mask teeth that are stained, chipped, or cracked. Veneers cover worn dentition and worn teeth, close gaps, and cover misshapen or otherwise damaged teeth that are in the smile zone. They can also make a person look younger and boost self-confidence. In short, veneers instantly provide a smile makeover. When I say instantly, I mean that the patients smile is completed in two to three weeks from start to finish.

In most cases involving veneers, I apply the veneers to teeth without doing any preliminary whitening to the actual teeth. In some cases, I know that a professional dental whitening will brighten the patient's teeth so much that I decide to do the whitening prior to performing a dental veneer procedure. In other words, when I whiten the underlying tooth structure, then I can apply more translucent veneers. It is optimal to have a whiter tooth structure before the veneer is applied. I tell patients that if they take care of their mouth with good oral hygiene, brushing, flossing, and regular dental cleaning appointments, the veneers should last for 15 to 20 years, or even longer.

PORCELAIN CROWNS

The cosmetic results of porcelain crowns have improved drastically over the years. However, they are a bit more invasive compared to Invisalign® or veneers. Porcelain crowns are a wonderful way to improve the smile and can do cosmetic wonders. They are indicated when there is an inherent health problem with a tooth, such as decay or a crack that has made it structurally unsound. The crown returns the tooth to a healthy state by making it stronger while giving the tooth a beautiful cosmetic appearance at the same time.

INVISALIGN®

Patients with crooked teeth, poorly shaped teeth, or over-lapped teeth are ideal candidates for Invisalign®. I always try to use the least invasive or conservative solution to meet the patient's goals and Invisalign® does just that. I put myself into my patient's shoes, imagining how I would want to be treated and how I would want the dentist to work on my teeth. Though many dentists use more aggressive procedures, common sense tells me that the least invasive method would be the best choice, provided it is one of the best methods to correct the problem. The Invisalign® treatment is anesthesia-free because the teeth themselves are not altered. It is a nice, discreet way to improve the smile.

Invisalign® has been used for approximately 15 years, and usage has increased during the last 10 years. Most adults can't stand the thought of metal in their mouth for two years, and Invisalign® eliminates the need for metal brackets and wires. Patients also love it because they can speak confidently when wearing the aligners. One of the best parts of Invisalign® for my patients is that they can take out the aligners whenever they want. At any moment, they can go from straightening their teeth to having nothing in their mouth. This may apply equally in a dating or a work-related situation.

With the Invisalign® treatment, teeth can be straightened without having any subsequent health problems for the gums. Brushing and flossing are not obstructed with the Invisalign® treatment because there are no obstructions in your mouth. Since there are no wires to brush through or floss around, the gum health (gingival health) remains stable during the course of treatment. Unlike with braces, the Invisalign® treatment allows you to eat whatever you want because there are no metal brackets and no wires to capture food. While it can be more expensive than traditional braces, Invisalign® usually is a quicker treatment than braces, while achieving the same result. The time frame of treatment can be anywhere from six months to three years.

Many of my patients can close minor gaps and spaces between their teeth with Invisalign® or porcelain veneers. For the larger space scenarios, I typically recommend a combination of Invisalign® followed by either composite bondings or porcelain veneers. The treatment really depends on the exact amount of space that needs to be closed. The size and shape of an individual's teeth also plays a huge role in deciding which route will give the best results. I often will initiate a cosmetic case by doing a partial Invisalign® treatment to close some of the larger gaps to more manageable spaces. Then I'll place six to eight porcelain veneers to achieve the perfect balance and proportionality of the teeth. A standard clear retainer is made and required to stabilize the end result for all cases involving the Invisalign® treatment. I do that because whenever the treatment plan involves Invisalign®, spaces may open up unless the patient wears a clear retainer at night to stabilize the teeth and keep them in their final positions.

GUM RESHAPING (AKA GINGIVAL RESHAPING)

I use the word "underrated" to describe the gums. In the world of cosmetic dentistry, the gums are often overlooked but play a huge role in achieving a gorgeous smile. When people think about a beautiful smile, they usually think, "teeth." Many people have straight, well-shaped, white teeth and yet their smile is still not beautiful. That is because the gum line around their front teeth is critical in completing that gorgeous smile. The teeth themselves can be picture perfect, yet without a proper gum line, the overall smile will just not look right in the end. There are two ways to reshape gums.

One way is to use a laser to contour the gums. In most of my cosmetic veneer cases, I enhance the smile by using a diode laser to give the gums the shape and level that they should have. In this non-invasive procedure, a laser is used to sculpt and reshape the gum tissues to achieve a balanced and pleasing aesthetic result. With the laser, patients usually experience no bleeding, no stitches, and very little anesthetic. Patients love that they absolutely feel no pain during this procedure or afterwards. This is normally a permanent solution for patients who practice good oral hygiene and get regular cleanings, though there can be relapses that necessitate touch-up work if patients don't take care of their teeth.

The second way to reshape the gums is with crown lengthening, which is a more invasive type of surgical procedure that typically requires a periodontist. For patients with a gummy smile, even if their teeth are the proper length, they often appear short because they are covered with too much gum tissue. For patients with mild or moderate gum irregularities, I consistently use laser-assisted gingival re-contouring to correct their smiles.

REPAIRING OLD, UGLY FILLINGS

The majority of people have old fillings in their mouths, which may be fine from a health standpoint, but they often look dark and unattractive. This can make people feel self-conscious when smiling, laughing, or simply talking. It is important for a dentist to evaluate if the old fillings are defective and need to be replaced. When a filling is old, a space may be created between the tooth and filling, allowing bacteria and food debris to enter the space, leading to tooth decay. Today, many state-of-the-art filling materials and procedures can leave a patient wondering which one of his or her teeth had the filling done on it. I can cosmetically blend the filling right in with the tooth and the surrounding teeth.

There are several options for replacing old, unattractive, and discolored fillings, beginning with white fillings or tooth-colored fillings. These can be matched so closely to the state of one's tooth that they are virtually indistinguishable. The second option is a porcelain crown. When a tooth is severely damaged, the entire tooth may need to be protected by placing a porcelain crown over it, which strengthens the patient's remaining tooth structure. A third option includes porcelain veneers. For patients with old fillings on their front teeth, I recommend porcelain veneers to give them that beautiful smile they desire, while correcting and eliminating the appearance of old fillings. When done properly using the best quality materials and techniques, veneers are very durable. They look natural and do not stain.

COSMETIC DENTAL WORK DOES NOT REQUIRE SPECIAL MAINTENANCE

Other than consistently wearing their retainers after an Invisalign® orthodontic treatment, I tell patients that maintenance on cosmetic dentistry is no different from maintenance without cosmetic dentistry. You need to brush in the morning, brush at night, floss once a day in the evening, and get regular dental cleanings. Patients will often ask, "What do I need to do to keep everything in the shape that it's in?" I tell them that there is nothing extra—"do what you would do prior to having the cosmetic procedure." There is no set of special requirements other than regular checkups, regular X-rays, regular cleanings, brushing, and flossing.

Many patients come into my office desiring a beautiful smile, though some have periodontal disease and a number of other issues. Decayed back teeth and missing teeth keep me from initiating any type of cosmetic enhancement on patients' front teeth. After all, the health of the mouth is the number one priority. For individuals, good dental hygiene is as important as cosmetics when it comes to their teeth. The overall health of their mouth is a priority, so any oral disease, tooth decay, or pathology needs to be eliminated prior to beginning cosmetic work.

(This content should be used for informational purposes only. It does not create a doctor-patient relationship with any reader and should not be construed as medical advice. If you need medical advice, please contact a doctor in your community who can assess the specifics of your situation.)